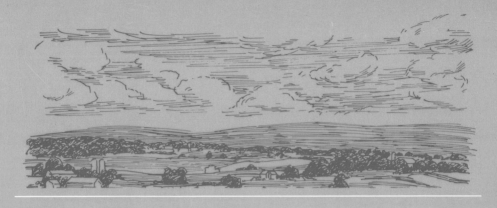

RURAL HEALTH ORGANIZATION

SOCIAL NETWORKS AND REGIONALIZATION

Edward W. Hassinger

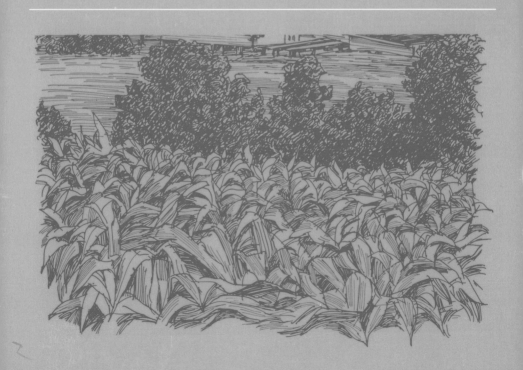

RURAL HEALTH ORGANIZATION

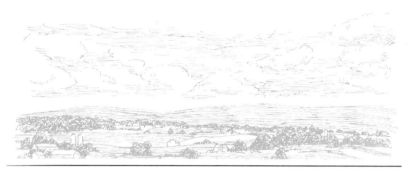

RURAL HEALTH ORGANIZATION

★ ★ ★

SOCIAL NETWORKS AND REGIONALIZATION

Edward W. Hassinger

IOWA STATE UNIVERSITY PRESS ● AMES, IOWA

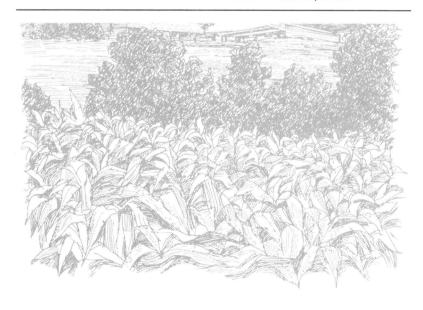

Edward W. Hassinger is professor of rural sociology at the University of Missouri-Columbia. He received the M.A. and Ph.D. degrees at the University of Minnesota.

Printed by The Iowa State University Press, Ames, Iowa 50010

First edition, 1982

Library of Congress Cataloging in Publication Data

Hassinger, Edward Wesley.
    Rural health organization.

    Includes bibliographical references and index.
    1. Rural health services—Administration. 2. Regional medical programs. I. Title. [DNLM: 1. Community health services—Organization and administration—United States. 2. Regional health planning—United States. 3. Rural health—United States. WA 541 AA1 H12r]
RA771.H35   362.1′0425   82-15323

ISBN 0-8138-1589-4   AACR2

TO MY WIFE ISABELLE

AND TO OUR CHILDREN
EDWARD, JR., JAMES, LOUISE, DIANE

CONTENTS

PREFACE

This monograph is an effort to place rural health services in a sociological and a societal context. I hope the approach will be useful to those who consider the problems of rural health care delivery in academia and those who formulate and implement policy. In discussing the organization of rural health services, I have described current programs that may become obsolete, but I have attempted to identify generalizations that transcend immediate programs and therefore hold promise for anticipating the future as well as understanding the past.

My debts are many with regard to this work. I have depended on a wide range of analysts and commentators. In many cases I have used their own words. My debt extends to my own department, the Department of Rural Sociology at the University of Missouri-Columbia, and its research mechanism, the Agricultural Experiment Station of the College of Agriculture-UMC. These organizations have supported research in rural health for almost four decades. This sociological effort, which predated medical sociology, originated with Charles E. Lively and was developed by Robert L. McNamara. I had the good fortune to work closely with McNamara and have continued this work in recent years in collaboration with Daryl J. Hobbs.

The writing of the manuscript was done under the sponsorship of the North Central Regional Center for Rural Development while I was on sabbatical leave at Iowa State University. I greatly appreciate the support of Ronald C. Powers, director of the Center, and Larry R. Whiting, editor for the Center. I also want to express my appreciation to the faculty, staff, and graduate students of the Department of Sociology and Anthropology at Iowa State University for their many kindnesses.

The final copy of the manuscript was typed by Melissa Baumann to whom I extend my personal thanks. Isabelle Cabaniss Hassinger read the manuscript for style and mechanics in all its stages. My debt to members of my family, to whom I have dedicated this book, is more than perfunctory.

RURAL HEALTH ORGANIZATION

Rural Society

It is commonly believed that rural areas are woefully deficient in health personnel and facilities and that consequently
the health status of rural people is poor. That belief is based
on four false or debatable points. First, treating rural society
as a uniform social entity is a fallacy. Second, there is little
evidence that the health status of rural people is worse than that
of urban people; it may even be better. Third, the belief that
health services are less accessible to rural than urban people may
be incorrect. And finally, it is not correct to equate availability or use of health services with health status--that is, we
cannot answer the question of whether or not rural health status
is inferior to urban health status by examining the relative
quantity of health services used by each.

This book discusses the organizational characteristics of
rural society that may affect the delivery of health services.
In particular it deals with the effects of informal group networks
and extralocal organizational relationships on the delivery of
health services in rural areas. These two areas tap very different aspects of community relationships, but each is extremely
important in understanding the delivery and utilization of contemporary rural health care.

This chapter presents a sketch of American rural society,
with emphasis on its heterogeneity. Rural sociologists generally
agonize over the definition of "rural" and the character of rural
society. Unable to separate rural from urban social systems in
terms of culture and organization, they nevertheless are unwilling
to abandon the distinction. After obligatory sparring, the census
definition of rural is usually accepted.

RURAL POPULATION

Rural Population according to the U.S. Census
The census definition of a rural population is those people
residing in places under 2,500 population and in the open country.

3

By this definition about 27 percent of the population of the
United States is rural. The rural population is subdivided into
persons residing on farms and those who do not. The rural nonfarm
population outnumbers the rural farm population by about seven to
one.

It is the farm population within the rural population category that has declined sharply. As late as 1920, the farm population was 32 million and represented 30 percent of the U.S. total.
By 1970, however, it was less than 10 million and represented 4.2
percent of the total. There is great diversity among the farms of
the nation. The smallest 22 percent (under 50 acres) have only
about 1 percent of the farmland, while the largest 3 percent
(2,000 acres and over) have about 46 percent. In 1977, 35 percent
of the farms had sales of less than $2,500, accounting for less
than 2 percent of the total sales, while 2 percent of the farms
had sales of $200,000 or more, accounting for 33 percent of the
sales (U.S. Bureau of the Census, 1978). It should be noted that
low agricultural sales by farm residents do not necessarily indicate low incomes for those families, because many have employment
off the farm. Nonfarm income is greater than farm income for a
majority of farm families.

The rural nonfarm population is even more diverse than the
rural farm population. It consists of people living in places of
under 2,500 population and in the open country but not on farms.
While we sometimes think of small town and rural nonfarm populations as synonymous, in fact less than one-third of the rural nonfarm population lives in small towns, while more than two-thirds
of it is in the open country but not on farms. Much of the rural
nonfarm and a considerable part of the farm population is in the
environs of metropolitan centers. It seems almost a contradiction
of terms to report that approximately 30 percent of the rural population is in metropolitan areas, but Calvin Beale finds that one
of the areas of greatest rural population surrounds the belt of
major cities from Washington, D.C., to New England and then west-
ward across the lower Great Lakes to southeastern Wisconsin.
"Here a majority of the rural people live within the bounds of
metropolitan areas and, although rural in residential setting,
often relate to the large cities for work or services. This area
has a sixth of our total rural population, and the number of rural
residents increased nearly half from 1940 to 1970" (Beale, 1978).

The principal criterion for designating an area as a Standard
Metropolitan Statistical Area (SMSA) is the presence of a city of
50,000 population or more. In such cases, the entire population
of the county in which the core city is located is counted as
metropolitan. In addition, contiguous counties may be designated
as metropolitan if they meet certain criteria establishing their
metropolitan character. Under this definition, metropolitan areas
contain rural as well as urban population.

The nonmetropolitan population, then, is quite different from
the rural population. Whereas the upper limit for places designated as rural is 2,499, places as large as 49,999 may be classi-

fied as nonmetropolitan. Places in the 25-50 thousand population range are likely to be important institutional centers and to offer services of considerable specialization. Analysts have wrestled with these population designations. One solution is to identify rural and urban populations *within* both the metropolitan and nonmetropolitan categories. An analysis by the U.S. Department of Agriculture divided counties into ten categories (see the details in the Appendix to this chapter) representing degrees of urbanness. It first places counties into metropolitan and nonmetropolitan categories. It then divides metropolitan counties on the basis of size of population and categorizes nonmetropolitan counties according to the number of residents and geographic proximity (adjacent or nonadjacent) to a metropolitan area (Hines et al., 1975). The most completely rural population is represented by a category of nonmetropolitan counties that has no urban population and is not adjacent to a metropolitan area. However, when this refinement is made, the category has only about 2 percent of the population of the United States and 8 percent of the rural population. Such refinements are not widely used in descriptive discourse because data relating to socioeconomic conditions (i.e., income, age, race) are not readily available for these categories and a ten-part classification is cumbersome.

Although it is easy to interchange rural and nonmetropolitan, the discussion of definitions makes it clear that rural/urban and nonmetropolitan/metropolitan are not equivalent categories. It also makes us aware that areas classified as rural or nonmetropolitan may vary considerably from our idealized perception of those terms. However, much of the available data are reported in these categories so it is prudent to be aware of their specifications and pitfalls. With this said, it must be acknowledged that the rural population has the characteristic of lower density and that the nonmetropolitan population is removed from the direct influence of larger centers. Furthermore, the rural/urban, nonmetropolitan/metropolitan categories show substantial differences on a wide range of socioeconomic variables from income to fertility (Duncan and Reiss, 1956; Hines et al., 1975).

Rural/Urban Population Trends
    The long-range trend has been for the rural population to decline as part of the U.S. total (from 95 percent in 1790 to 27 percent in 1970). This has resulted from a sharp reduction in the farm segment of the rural population. Meanwhile, the rural nonfarm population has increased in number and as a percentage of the total population since 1920 (farm and nonfarm population were first reported separately in 1920). It is of considerable interest that in the census period 1970-1980, for the first time since 1790 (in what has been called the urban to rural population turnaround), the rural population increased as a proportion of the U.S. total. While much of the growth of rural population is in or around metropolitan areas, growth also extends to more rural areas (Beale, 1978).

Diversity in Socioeconomic Characteristics
     It is worthwhile to consider some of the diversity within
the rural and/or nonmetropolitan population categories.

Age. The median age of nonmetropolitan and metropolitan populations is similar. Yet if one identifies counties of highest and
lowest median age, virtually all of them are nonmetropolitan.
That is, some nonmetropolitan counties have the oldest populations
in the country, while other nonmetropolitan counties have the
youngest.

Income. Rural areas have higher rates of poverty than urban
areas. Not only level of employment but also level of remunera-
tion account for the high level of rural poverty. Many workers
are underemployed, employed less than full time, or are poorly
compensated for their work.
     Poverty is chronic in some rural areas, including those with
substantial minorities in the South and Southwest as well as those
without substantial minorities as in Appalachia, the Ozarks, and
the Northern Cutover.
     In spite of these realities, it would be incorrect to regard
rural populations as uniformly deprived. The rate of industrial
employment has increased faster in rural than in urban areas.
Farm income, although variable from year to year, is generally
increasing. Some rural areas have experienced boom times in the
exploitation of natural resources. As with other socioeconomic
variables, there is great diversity in the income of people within
rural communities as well as between rural areas and communities.

Occupation. Although farming is prominently associated with rural
society, farm employment is a minor occupation in nonmetropolitan
America. For example, in 1970 only 8.5 percent of the nonmetropolitan labor force was employed in agriculture (farmers, farm
managers, and hired farm laborers), while 36 percent were white-
collar workers and 33 percent were craftsmen and operatives.

Minorities. Black Americans have migrated in large numbers from
the rural south to metropolitan areas. Today the black population
is more urban than the white. The rural black population, however, is still heavily concentrated in the South.
     The second largest minority in the United States is Mexican-
American. Mexican-Americans are concentrated in five southwestern
states. Although many find employment in agriculture as hired
laborers, they are likely to reside in urban areas.
     Native Americans are the most rural of major minority groups.
Rural Native Americans are concentrated on reservations, where
some of the greatest economic deprivation in the United States
prevails.
     Other minorities with strong rural identities that contribute
to the diversity of the rural population include the French-speak-
ing Cajuns of southern Louisiana and religious communities such as
the Amish and Hutterites.

Isolation of Rural Populations

Although distance and/or physical features of the land iso-
late some rural people from certain services, we too readily
assume that isolation is the condition of all rural people. The
settlement patterns of rural America vary from place to place. In
the Midwest, for example, land is divided in a checkerboard fashion with farmsteads quite evenly distributed and trade centers at
short, regular intervals. In the western plains, ranches thin
out, settlement is concentrated along major transportation routes,
and there are extensive outback areas of sparse settlements and
limited services. In the Appalachian Mountains, the rural population may be clustered in limited spaces along the "hollers," with
scattered population away from the valleys. In eastern states, by
contrast, rural people may be concentrated on the fringes of metropolitan centers to which they commute for employment. Conditions of isolation exist, but isolation is not a universal or
even predominant rural condition.

Technology has contributed immensely to the reduction of
rural isolation. Historically, roads and railroads connected
remote areas to markets. The development and common use of the
automobile and truck freed rural people from their dependence on
trade centers within a "team haul." Almost no area is without
telephone service and television reception. Today even the most
remote locations benefit from highly sophisticated communication
technology through use of satellites.

VALUES AND BELIEFS OF RURAL PEOPLE

A question that has long intrigued rural sociologists is
whether or not there is a unique set of rural values and/or beliefs. Olaf Larson's answer to the question in 1978 was different
than it was in 1964 when he and Everett Rogers wrote, "Rural-urban
differences in values are decreasing as America moves in the direction of mass society" (Larson and Rogers, 1964). The data he
has examined since then (much of it from Gallup polls) led him to
"challenge any assumption that all the important rural-urban differences in values and beliefs are rapidly vanishing, if they
have not already been obliterated by the forces of a mass society"
(Larson, 1978). Larson comments on the diversity within rural
America and observes that rural society shares in the strains and
tensions of the larger society. Norval Glenn and Jon Alston also
compared farmers and other occupational categories using data from
Gallup polls from 1953 to 1965. They found that significant differences existed and that they were in the expected direction.
Farmers, when compared with other occupational groups, were more
prejudiced, less favorable to civil liberties, less tolerant of
deviance, more ethnocentric and isolationist, more work oriented,
and more puritanical (Glenn and Alston, 1967).

Differences in values or beliefs between rural and urban populations are differences of degree rather than kind and tend to be
quite small. There is danger in magnifying these differences into
separate value systems—one for rural society, the other for urban

society. The diversity of values and beliefs of rural people
noted by Larson argues against this interpretation. In addition,
if the purpose is to use rural/urban differences in values and
beliefs to account for differences in health behavior, one should
be aware that beliefs are not a very good predictor of health
behavior (Battistella, 1968; Weisenberg et al., 1980). It is part
of the general failure in social research to find much correspondence between what people say and believe and what they do
(LaPiere, 1934; Deutscher, 1966).

In spite of these misgivings, the idea of rural and urban
differences that relate to behavior (eventually to health behavior) need not be abandoned. Instead, organizational characteristics of rural society that distinguish it from urban society
should be considered and their relationships to rural health
behavior should be explored. Values and beliefs appear to be most
useful as predictors of health behavior when viewed within the
context of primary group relations. Gary Fine and Sherryl Kleinman (1979) say, "Individuals within the affective boundaries of
the interlocking group's network who have identifications with the
subcultural population are most committed to the subculture."
Thus beliefs are part of the ongoing social process that finds
definition and support in primary groups.

ORGANIZATION OF RURAL SOCIETY: THE RURAL COMMUNITY
The community is the most inclusive social unit below the
society as a whole. It is an area in which groups and individuals
interact in the everyday affairs of making a living, socializing
members, maintaining social control, providing opportunities for
social participation, and caring for those in need and in crisis
situations (Warren, 1978). The essence of community is the interaction of groups and individuals in patterned relationships as
they pursue these activities within local settings. While there
is some opinion to the contrary, most discussions regard the community as a limited geographical area with more or less defined
boundaries.

The beginning of rural sociology is often marked by the
publication in 1915 of Charles Galpin's *The Social Anatomy of an
Agricultural Community*. In it he delineated the service relationships of trade centers and open-country populations of a rural
Wisconsin county. On the basis of the identifying centers where
open-country populations obtain dry goods and groceries he constructed service area maps of the county and called the trade
center and its service area the basic community area (Galpin,
1915).

The most common nonmetropolitan settlement pattern in the
United States is a concentration of people in trade centers (villages, towns, small cities), with associated hinterlands more
sparsely settled by agricultural workers on farmsteads and other
open-country residents. When Galpin and other early rural sociologists were making their observations, trade centers tended to be

located at fairly regular intervals, reflecting the time-distance
that residents of the open country could conveniently travel in a
day for trade and service activities from the outer reaches of the
area and back. In the days of the "team-haul," centers were located about eight to ten miles apart with a radius of about four
to five miles from the center of the periphery. With changes in
transportation and aspirations of rural people, the service relationships of rural areas have been altered. Trade centers no
longer can claim an exclusive trade territory and a loyal clientele. However, instead of trade centers simply being spread farther apart, they have become more specialized, offering different
kinds of services, which suggests a division of labor and a hierarchical ordering among them from simple to complex within an
expanded area. The core of the expanded service community is a
dominant place (often referred to as a growth center), which is a
point of centralization for activities of the larger community and
a place of population concentration.

    Karl Fox developed a conceptual overlay of the larger commu-
nity, which he designated as Functional Economics Areas (FEAs)
(Fox and Kumar, 1966). Under midwestern conditions, an FEA,
according to Fox, would consist of a central place of perhaps
25,000 people or more, a number of surrounding retail and convenience centers, and an open-country population. The area of influence would depend both on the size of the central place and the
population density of the surrounding area. Again, under midwestern conditions, such an area would contain about 5,000 square
miles or from eight to ten counties--approximately a 60-minute
commuting radius from the periphery to the center. Such an area
would include all but the most specialized services and would en-
compass an economy sufficient to provide employment within the
area. Furthermore, Fox regards FEAs as principal units for planning and policy implementation.

    One can hardly overlook the parallel between the city with
its differentiated economic activities and land use and the larger
nonmetropolitan community with its commercial core, differentiated
pattern of service, and population concentrations in the hinterland. It should not stretch one's imagination much to view the
larger rural community as a city which often includes the production of food and fiber in biological factories.

    It is now common to divide the relationships of groups and
individuals that take place within the community and those in
which local people relate to those outside the community. Following Roland Warren (1978), relationships of the first type are
referred to as horizontal and the second type as vertical.

Horizontal Relationships

    At the base of the rural/urban difference in horizontal rela-
tions is the difference in population density. Since the time of
Emile Durkheim (1893; trans. ed. 1964) population density has been
regarded as positively associated with the specialization and for-
mality of social organizations characteristic of cities. The

obverse of this is that the lower population density of rural communities yields more homogeneity and greater informality in social
relationships. In rural communities, informal groups such as
families, cliques, and neighborhoods are especially prominent.
Patterns of relationships based on informal groups grow over time
and form natural support systems that are quite intricate. They
are also fragile and subject to disruptions by outside influences.
Informality in rural communities extends to task-oriented groups
such as school, church, and local government, all of which are
likely to be conducted on a "friends and neighbors" basis. Chapter Three presents a more detailed discussion of informal social
structures in the community. It is especially pertinent to health
behavior since health beliefs and health decisions are often vali-
dated by informal groups, and informal group networks provide
referral and support mechanisms in the utilization of health services. Informal support networks in rural communities may be as
effective in accounting for rural/urban differences in the use of
health services as are differences in the availability of health
services.

Vertical Relationships
        Some writers regard the crucial organizational problem of
American rural society to be its linkage with the larger society
(Vidich and Bensman, 1958; Warren, 1978). Rural communities in
the United States are connected in numerous ways with the larger
society. There is the common source of entertainment and information from television and other mass communications. But rural
structures are related to the larger society more precisely than
that. For example, local schools have vertical relationships
with elements of the state and federal educational bureaucracies
that directly affect the characteristics of local school systems.
        In parallel manner, local health services are affected by the
health bureaucracies. Even a small community hospital, for
example, is enmeshed in a bewildering array of linkages. Sydney
Croog and Donna VerSteeg (1972) cite as a partial list 15 national
and 15 state agencies with which hospitals may interact. At the
national level are such units as the Department of Health and
Human Services (formerly the Department of Health, Education and
Welfare) and its administration of Medicare through the Social
Security Administration; the Joint Commission on Accreditation of
Hospitals; and the Department of Justice, Bureau of Narcotics. At
the state level, hospitals might be expected to interact with
agencies of licensure, reimbursement (i.e., Blue Cross, Medicaid),
and planning. In addition to the governmental and professional
agencies and associations Croog and VerSteeg listed, hospitals
deal with commercial suppliers, public and private granting agencies, labor unions, and insuring (i.e., malpractice) agencies
among others. The federal government's participation in reimbursement through Medicare imposes far-reaching requirements dealing with certification, fiscal record keeping, quality review procedures, and facility expansion (within the planning framework).

Similarly, other units of the local health care system such as
physicians, dentists, laboratories, and nursing homes have numerous extralocal connections.
    The relationship between local and extralocal organizations
is not likely to be between equals. Rather, the outside organization is likely to be a bureaucracy of power and reach not matched
by local organizations. The bureaucracies of mass society require
a certain quality of performance and accountability from their
local connections. Local organizations of some size and resources
are more compatible with these needs than are individuals and
organizations of very limited resources. At the very least, the
local organization must be able to keep records and communicate
with the central agency.
    Regionalization is a concept especially pertinent to a dis-
cussion of linkages between local and extralocal structures. It
is notable that the federal government has attempted to coordinate
activities in many areas. The most comprehensive effort is
through multipurpose substate units. These units take the form of
councils of governments (COGs) or regional planning commissions
(RPCs). In 1978, there were 555 area-wide units covering 2,724
counties and embracing 96 percent of the population of the United
States. The formation of multicounty substate units is virtually
assured since approval by them is a requirement for funding of
some 240 federal programs (Stam, 1979). The federal government
regards the clearinghouse function of local government councils
as a form of decentralization--federal agencies sharing decision
making with local units. However, from the community perspective,
this process represents centralization of decision making.
    Early attempts at regionalization of health services were
voluntary. The first systematic program was in the 1930s in
Maine, where the Bingham Associates Fund established a regional
program between hospitals in small towns in Maine and a medical
center in Boston (Roemer, 1976a). Another early voluntary effort
often cited as a model for regionalization of hospital services is
the Rochester Regional Hospital Council, which subsequently
extended its influence to an 11-county area.
    Most of the health planning programs today are channeled
through special-purpose agencies rather than general clearinghouse
substate agencies such as local government councils. The National
Health Planning and Resources Development Act of 1974 (P.L.
93-641) is the principal federal program for health services planning. Among the priorities of the act (Sec. 1502) is "the development of multi-institutional systems for coordination or consolidation of institutional health services (including obstetrics,
pediatrics, emergency medical, intensive and coronary care, and
radiation therapy services)," which is a statement of regionalization.
    In the organization of rural health services, the tension
between local and centralized organizations (and the controls this
implies) is a constant theme. However, even though bureaucratic
centers tend to dominate the relationships, organizations of rural

communities need not be passive. Nor, as the diversity of rural
society suggests, are the relationships uniform. As this discussion develops, the two principal topics will be the informal
patterns of local control in health behaviors and the linkages of
local and centralized health organizations through regionalization.

APPENDIX

Residence Classification according to Degree of
Urban/Rural Influence

      In total, the ten groups of counties (four metropolitan, six
nonmetropolitan) represent varying degrees of urban influence upon
the counties' populations--the groupings represent an urban/rural
dimension with the most urban being the core counties of greater
metropolitan areas and the most rural being nonmetropolitan
counties with no urban residents and not adjacent to a Standard
Metropolitan Statistical Area (SMSA).

  I. Metropolitan (SMSA) counties
      A. Greater metropolitan--counties of SMSAs having at least
          1 million population in 1970 (175 counties). Examples
          are New York City, Chicago, and Los Angeles.
          1. Core counties--counties containing the primary cen-
              tral city of greater metropolitan areas (48 coun-
              ties). Examples are Cook County, Illinois; the 5
              counties of New York City; and St. Louis City and
              County.
          2. Fringe counties--suburban counties of greater metro-
              politan areas (127 counties). Examples are Mont-
              gomery County, Maryland; Fairfax County, Virginia (of
              the Washington, D.C., metropolitan area); and Bucks
              County, Pennsylvania (of the Philadelphia metropoli-
              tan area).
      B. Medium metropolitan--these counties are SMSAs of 250,000
          to 999,999 population (258 counties). Some SMSAs that
          fall into this category include Phoenix, Oklahoma City,
          Madison, Birmingham, and Salt Lake City.
      C. Small metropolitan--these counties are SMSAs of less than
          250,000 population (179 counties). Examples include
          Portland, Maine; Eugene, Oregon; and Hamilton-Middletown,
          Ohio.
 II. Nonmetropolitan (non-SMSA) counties
      A. Urbanized adjacent--counties contiguous to SMSAs and hav-
          ing an aggregate urban population of at least 20,000 res-
          idents (191 counties).
      B. Urbanized not adjacent--counties not contiguous to SMSAs
          and having an aggregate urban population of at least
          20,000 inhabitants (137 counties).

C. Less urbanized adjacent--counties contiguous to SMSAs and
    having an aggregate urban population of 2,500 to 19,999
    inhabitants (564 counties).
D. Less urbanized not adjacent--counties not contiguous to
    SMSAs and having an aggregate urban population of 2,500
    to 19,999 inhabitants (721 counties).
E. Totally rural adjacent--counties contiguous to SMSAs and
    having no urban population (246 counties).
F. Totally rural not adjacent--counties not contiguous to
    SMSAs and having no urban population (626 counties)
    (Hines et al., 1975).

CHAPTER 2

Health Services
and Health Status

The American people have developed a complex and sophisticated health care system. The crucial question in any consideration of health services or health behavior is the health status of
the populations involved. But health status is a complex concept
and partly a matter of definition. Level of health most certainly
cannot be equated to the quantity of health services in an area
whether urban or rural.

HEALTH PERSONNEL
    In the United States the physician is the focus of personal
health care. Alternatives that exist are on the fringes of legitimacy. Associated with physicians, however, is a complex system
of health services that includes other health professionals and
technicians, hospitals, nursing homes, and elaborate technology
for diagnosis, treatment, and rehabilitation. The patterning
and relationships of these personnel and facilities represent the
organization of the health care delivery system.

Physicians
    There are over 435,000 medical doctors (MDs) and about
15,000 doctors of osteopathy (DOs) in the United States. Most of
them are in office-based practices, but an increasing number are
full-time staff members or residents-in-training at hospitals.
The following is a tabulation of the major professional activities
of MDs in 1978 (Glandon and Shapiro, 1980).

Total physicians (MDs)	437,486
Physicians in patient care	342,714
Office-based practice	239,866
Hospital-based practice	102,848
Residents	60,610
Full-time staff	42,238
Other professional activity	33,097
Medical teaching	7,025

15

Administration	11,858
Research	11,437
Other	2,777
Unclassified and inactive	61,675

Specialization is one of the most apparent characteristics of physicians. Of the physicians in patient care, only 16 percent were in general or family practice in 1978. Areas of specialization with large numbers were: internal medicine (16 percent), general surgery (9 percent), psychiatry (7 percent), obstetrics and gynecology (7 percent), and pediatrics (6 percent) (Glandon and Shapiro, 1980). About one-half the physicians in the United States are board-certified by one of the 22 American specialty boards.

For decades, commentators have worried about a shortage of doctors. The shortage has been alleviated through an increase of physicians trained in American medical schools and by an influx of graduates of foreign medical schools. In the decade from 1965 to 1975, 25 new medical schools were established and the size of classes in existing schools was increased substantially. As a consequence, the number of first-year medical students more than doubled from 1960 to 1975--from 7,000 to 14,874. In addition, an influx of foreign medical graduates began in the 1950s. In 1975, foreign graduates accounted for 44 percent of all newly licensed physicians and today they represent about one-fifth of the physicians practicing in the United States. Efforts are being made to curb the number of foreign graduates, and the large expansion in number of medical schools and class size has also ended. Although federal support for medical education expansion has ceased, entrance to medical schools remains competitive and it is unlikely that enrollment will fall below capacity in the foreseeable future.

While the number of physicians and the capacity of the training facilities suggest that the physician shortage has ended, problems remain with availability of primary-care physicians and distribution of physicians. Efforts have been made to increase the number of primary-care physicians through the federal government's capitation support to medical schools. In family practice, one of the newer specialty boards (established in 1970), the number of approved residency programs increased from 49 in 1970 to 288 in 1977 and the number of residents from 290 in 1970 to 4,675 in 1976.

Physicians are distributed unevenly by region of the country and especially by metropolitan and nonmetropolitan divisions. The New England, Middle Atlantic, and Pacific states have the most favorable physician/population ratios, while the east south central, west south central, and west north central states have the least favorable. There are about five times as many people for each physician in the smallest nonmetropolitan counties as there are in the largest metropolitan counties (USDHEW, 1976b). Of con-

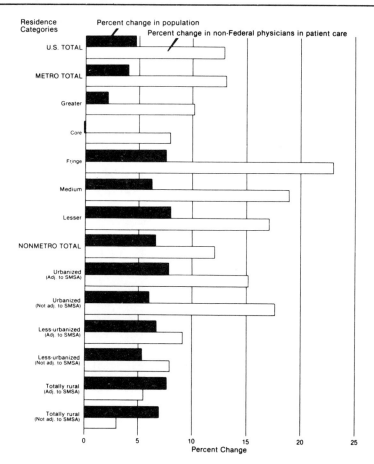

Fig. 2.1.   Changes in population and supply of physicians by
residence, 1970-1975.   (Ahearn, 1979)

siderable interest is the fact that metropolitan areas are receiving more than their proportionate share of the increase in physicians (Fig. 2.1).

Other Health Personnel
      Physicians represent only about 6 percent of the 6.7 million
people employed in the health services industry (USDHEW, 1980).
Most of these workers are engaged in activities that support physicians, as demonstrated by the fact that more than one-half of
them are employed in hospitals.
      Of the health professionals, nurses are most numerous. Over
1.1 million registered nurses were employed in 1978 (USDHEW,
1980). Practical nurses, nursing aides, orderlies, and attendants

constituted an additional 1.4 million health services employees.
Health technologists and technicians numbered almost 500,000 and
therapists another 200,000 (USDHEW, 1980).

Nonphysician practitioners, including physician assistants
and nurse practitioners, have become increasingly important in the
delivery of health services, especially in rural areas. Their
role in the health care delivery system will be explored later.

Chiropractors are the most visible alternative to established
medical practitioners. Their philosophy and therapy differ substantially from mainstream medicine. About 17,000 chiropractors
practice in the nation, most of them in solo practice or in
association with one or two others. Little specialization or
referral of patients occurs within the profession.

ORGANIZATION OF MEDICAL PRACTICE

Trends in Solo Practice
        As noted earlier, most physicians have office-based practices.
The traditional organization of practice was for individual physicians, with limited support personnel, to establish a practice
among a loyal clientele in the simple setting of an examining room.
The trend today is toward a more complex organization of the
delivery of health services. Even if physicians remain in solo
practice, and fewer are doing so, their practices are likely to
employ more support personnel, use more laboratory facilities, and
focus more on hospitals. The locations of physicians' offices,
whether in rural or urban communities, are likely to be near hospitals and in urban areas clustered with many other doctors in
medical buildings. Thus physicians today are almost certain to
practice in workshop settings where they are able to control tim-
ing of work and interpersonal relationships. The workshop may be
an office suite of a solo practitioner, a group clinic, a hospital,
or similar facilities or combinations of facilities. Among the
characteristics of the workshop are: a place of service is continually available to clients; investment can be made in heavy and
immobile equipment; tasks can be subdivided utilizing personnel of
different skills and different skill levels; more than one job can
be taken at a time, thus work is not turned away and the server
does not wait between jobs; clients are guests. which reinforces
the server's control; quality of performance and time requirements
are more easily concealed from clients; and "dirty work" and
"clean work" are more easily segregated (Goffman, 1961).

Group Practice
        There is a growing trend toward group practice. However,
many of the groups are small, differing only slightly from solo or
partnership practices. Others are complex organizations with
extensive support personnel and facilities, including hospitals.
Distinctions are commonly made between single specialty, multispecialty, and family practice groups and between those that offer
prepayment plans to clients and those that do not.

A 1975 survey by the American Medical Association (AMA) reported that 24 percent of the nonfederal physicians in the United States were in 8,483 group practices. The AMA's definition of group medical practice is medical service by three or more physicians formally organized to provide medical care, consultation, diagnosis and/or treatment, through the joint use of equipment and personnel, and with income from medical practice distributed in accordance with methods previously determined by members of the group (AMA, 1977). Fifty-nine percent of the group physicians practiced in single specialty groups, 35 percent in multispecialty groups, and 6 percent in family practice groups. About 8 percent of the group practices, involving about 20 percent of the physicians in group practice, provided some care on a prepaid basis.

The average size of medical groups was 7.9 physicians. Multispecialty groups averaged 13.2, single specialty groups 5.1, and family practice groups 4.4 physicians. Nonprepaid groups were smaller than prepaid groups--averaging 6.9 and 19.0 physicians respectively (Goodman et al., 1976).

Using these data, Barry Eisenberg (1977) compared the characteristics of group medical practice in metropolitan and nonmetropolitan areas. Of the medical group practices identified in the survey, 81 percent were located in metropolitan areas and 19 percent in nonmetropolitan areas. Nonmetropolitan group practices averaged 6.6 physicians compared with 8.2 physicians in metropolitan group practices. Nonmetropolitan groups were more likely than metropolitan groups to be family practice or multispecialty groups, while metropolitan groups were more likely to be single specialty (Table 2.1).

Group practices in nonmetropolitan areas tended to provide more auxiliary services such as laboratory and X-ray services.

Although the number of group practices increased between 1969 and 1975, 25 percent of those present in 1969 did not survive to 1975. Differences of abandonment in metropolitan compared to nonmetropolitan locations were slight. Freshnock and Goodman (1979) concluded that internal factors such as size of group and presence of a business administrator were more important to survival than were external factors such as change in population density and physician/population ratios.

Health Maintenance Organizations

One type of prepaid group practice in particular has gained public attention and some support from the federal government. Generally known as Health Maintenance Organizations (HMOs), these groups represent not only an alternative way of financing health services but also an alternative method of organizing them. HMOs

Table 2.1. Distribution of group practices in metropolitan and nonmetropolitan areas, 1975

Type of practice	Percent of groups in each type practice	
	Metropolitan	Nonmetropolitan
Family practice	7.2	25.1
Single specialty	60.5	28.4
Multispecialty	32.3	46.5

contract with a defined population of clients to provide comprehensive health services for a fixed per capita fee. Health services usually include all physician services; inpatient and outpatient hospital services such as immunizations and periodic
physical examinations are emphasized. The claim is made that the
HMO model should reduce costs because physicians benefit economically from keeping costs low and therefore will encourage preventive measures and discourage unneeded surgery or hospitalization
(Luft, 1980). A leading advocate of HMOs, Paul M. Ellwood, Jr.,
believes that this form of organization will bring health care
services into the competitive marketplace. He says that competition over prices and benefits would be encouraged and monopolies
would be discouraged. HMOs would expand or fail depending on the
judgment of clients in the marketplace (Ellwood, 1974).

It is probably no accident that HMOs have had a great impact
on the delivery of health services in the Minnesota twin cities,
Minneapolis and St. Paul, where Ellwood is president of Inter-
study, a health policy study group. In that area, seven HMOs compete for clients and about 14 percent of the population is enrolled
in HMO programs.

The largest and best known of the HMOs, and often regarded as
a prototype, is the Kaiser-Permanente Medical Care Program. The
program was founded for Kaiser shipyard workers on the West Coast
during World War II. It is now found in California, Oregon,
Hawaii, Ohio, and Colorado. Kaiser-Permanente has a medical staff
of about 2,000 and 24 hospitals with about 5,000 beds for more
than 2 million enrolled members.

The federal government sought to encourage HMOs through
legislation in 1973 that provided funds for feasibility studies
as well as for planning and start-up. However, because of excessive services required by federal guidelines, few HMOs were
established as a result of this legislation. Amendments to the
legislation in 1976 permitted greater flexibility and gave impetus
to the formation of new HMOs. On the basis of a survey conducted
in 1977, it was estimated that about 6.5 million persons were
enrolled in HMO-type programs (Metropolitan Life Insurance Co.,
1978).

Neighborhood Health Centers
Another organizational model for delivery of comprehensive
medical services to a geographically defined population is the
Neighborhood Health Center (NHC). Established as a program of
the Economic Opportunity Act of 1964, NHCs were designed to make
a broad range of health services accessible under one roof and to
deliver comprehensive health services to residents of low income
areas. Major emphasis is on ambulatory services, health-related
supportive services, and outreach programs. Community laypersons
are involved in policy making. While NHCs are most often associated with low income urban areas, they are also found in rural
areas.

HOSPITALS
     Hospitals are vital in the organization of medical practices
from solo office-based practices to those of prestigious medical
centers. Hospitals exemplify division of labor and organizational
ability to focus a number of specialists and personnel with a wide
range of skills on the task of treating and caring for patients.
Anne Somers (1971a, b) views the hospital as the organizational
center of the health care delivery system. The American Hospital
Association put forward a plan which would establish 400 "Health
Care Corporations" responsible for health maintenance, primary
and specialty care, and rehabilitation care within a defined area.
Known as the Ameriplan, it makes hospitals the organizational foci
of the local systems.
     There are a number of ways of classifying hospitals: general
and special; short term and long term; federal and nonfederal;
public, nonprofit-voluntary, and proprietary. General medical
and surgical hospitals, which are commonly regarded as community
hospitals, range in size from under 50 to 1,000 beds or more. Of
the more than 1 million general hospital beds, over two-thirds
are nonprofit-voluntary or proprietary. There are about 4.3 nonfederal general hospital beds per 1,000 population. Hospitals of
size often have outpatient clinics, and emergency rooms are increasingly access points to the medical care system. Specialty
hospitals are often long-term facilities. Almost 1 in 4 of all
hospital beds are devoted to psychiatric care and are likely to be
government supported.
     Hospital facilities are more equitably divided between rural
and urban areas than physicians' services (Table 2.2). This is

Table 2.2. Short-term community hospital facilities
            per 100,000 population by area, 1975

Population area	Facilities	Beds
	(number per 100,000)	
Metropolitan	2	460
Greater	2	459
Core	2	519
Fringe	2	329
Medium	2	447
Lesser	2	502
Nonmetropolitan	5	428
Urbanized		
Adjacent	3	379
Nonadjacent	4	582
Less urbanized		
Adjacent	5	393
Nonadjacent	7	487
Totally rural		
Adjacent	6	268
Nonadjacent	9	333
U.S. total	3	451

Source: Ahearn, 1979
Note: The original data came from USDHEW, 1976a.

due mainly to federal support, which favored hospital construction
in rural areas. Many of the rural hospitals are small and have
difficulty maintaining quality medical staff and adequate bed
censuses. Like other aspects of rural life, there are influences
toward consolidation of rural hospitals while at the same time
local communities strongly resist closing their hospitals.

HEALTH STATUS
     Here is an old question: are rural or urban people healthier?
That the question has not been answered to everyone's satisfaction
indicates that health status is difficult to measure. It also
indicates that differences between the health statuses of rural
and urban people are not great enough to overwhelm the crudeness
of defining and measuring health status. While some might see
this as an argument for greater refinement in technique, others
might conclude that such fine differences make little practical
difference.
     What are health and sickness? A common definition of health
is provided by the World Health Organization as "a state of complete physical, mental and social well-being, and not merely the
absence of disease or infirmity." Compared to such an ideal situation, everyone would be in a state of nonhealth to some degree.
According to Andrew Twaddle and Richard Hessler (1977), nonhealth
conditions are labeled disease, illness, and sickness--terms that
although often used interchangeably are given distinct meaning by
these authors.
     Disease has a biological referent. "One organism invades
another with predictable, negatively valued outcomes for the host,
or there is a breakdown in the anatomical structure of an orga-
nism." Diagnosis by physicians is the identification and labeling
of disease statuses.
     Illness is a subjective feeling of nonhealth by the affected
person. The basis for illness may be disease, but it may also
occur in the absence of disease   The perception of illness may
prompt a person to seek professional consultation or self-treatment. Illness is classified as a sociopsychological status.
     Sickness is a social status and the unique province of socio-
logical analysis. Sociological discussions of nonhealth depend
heavily on the view that incumbency in the sick status (the sick
role) represents a deviation from normal social obligations (working, going to school, performing household tasks) because of illness.

The Sick Role Concept
     Persons identified as sick are not only permitted but expected
to assume a socially defined status and act in accordance with it.
They may assume the sick role by claiming illness, but confirmation
depends on concurrence by significant others (e.g., children by
parents; peers by peers), and physicians are the "great legiti-
mizers" of the sick role.

Two privileges and two obligations are usually associated with the sick role (Parsons, 1951).

• Sick persons are exempted from normal obligations (going to school, shoveling the sidewalk, going to work, etc.).
• Sick persons are not held personally responsible for their condition.
• There is an obligation by sick persons to attempt to overcome their illness.
• There is an obligation, except for minor illness, by sick persons to seek competent help.

Thus in exchange for the privileges of exemption from normal obligations and dispensation from personal blame, sick persons remove themselves as quickly as possible, and in an acceptable manner, from the sick (deviant) status. Society, for its part, provides substantial resources to help persons avoid (through prevention) or escape (through treatment and rehabilitation) the sick role. Social monitoring is also part of the process of entering and remaining in the sick role. Much of this monitoring is informal and depends on sanctions of family and friends. Also, professionals stand at the gates of the medical care system and judge sick role status as a condition for entrance.

The sick role, so defined, is obviously an ideal type and some disease/illness conditions do not lend themselves exactly to it. Chronic disease is one such important category. Chronic diseases are, by definition, long-term conditions for which there is no likelihood of complete cure, thus offering low possibility of escape from the sick role. However, the goal of treatment in chronic ailments such as heart disease, diabetes, and cancer is return to normal activities.

The sick role for alcoholics is even more problematic. It is not certain that society is willing to set aside personal blame, consider it a disease, and offer treatment instead of incarceration. Alcoholics for their part may not accept the obligations of the sick role, especially to seek competent assistance (Orcutt and Cairl, 1979).

The trend has been to spread the net of sickness over a wider area to include not only such conditions as mental illness and alcoholism but other behaviors that have traditionally been regarded as delinquent. While this seems like a humane approach, there may be abuses—as when dissident behavior is labeled mental illness. Furthermore, the sick role may be counterproductive for those with behavior problems because it absolves them from personal responsibility for their conditions and thus deprives them of a means of altering it.

Persons are increasingly being held responsible for failing to take precautions or for practicing a life-style that leads to illness. For example, in an analysis of 2,238 cases selected from 42,880 discharges in six contrasting hospital populations in and around Boston for the year 1976, relatively few patients accounted

for a large amount of costs; thus the high-cost 13 percent of the
patients consumed as many resources as the low-cost 87 percent.
The researchers emphasized the point that adverse life-styles were
more prevalent in the medical records of high-cost patients.
Alcoholism, heavy smoking, and obesity were particularly prominent
among the high-cost patients. The authors apparently do not hold
these high-cost patients blameless when they suggest that "preventive incentives through insurance or health taxes on selected
hazardous habits (or commodities that they consume) may deserve
careful attention in any debate on national health insurance"
(Zook and Moore, 1980).
     The concept of the sick role has been subject to a great deal
of critical comment, including the extreme point of view that it
should be abandoned as a conceptual basis for analysis (Berkanovic,
1972; Segall, 1976; Levine and Kozloff, 1978). A value of the
sick role is that it establishes a sociological framework for the
analysis of nonhealth conditions As an ideal type, its usefulness is not lost if behavior does not conform precisely to one or
another of its components. Rather, it helps distinguish between
classes of diseases and populations in their nonhealth behavior.
For example, one might hypothesize that significant others in the
rural setting would condemn alcoholism on moral grounds to a
greater extent than their urban counterparts (Lowe and Peek,
1974). Thus on the "personal blame" dimension, rural persons
would be less likely to gain sick role incumbency for this condition.

Data Pertaining to the Sick Role
     There is no general body of data that identifies incumbents
of the sick role. However, of the general indices available,
reports of acute illnesses and disability days are the closest
approximations. These data are available from the Health Inter-
view Survey (HIS) of the National Health Survey. The HIS is based
on information from a continuing nationwide random sample of
households that yields interviews with about 116,000 persons in
40,000 households per year. Disability days are classified into
days of restricted activity (a day in which a person cuts down on
his usual activities because of an illness or injury), bed disability days, or work-loss days. The data in the HIS reports are
presented by metropolitan and nonmetropolitan categories, with the
nonmetropolitan category divided for nonfarm and farm populations.
     Acute illnesses are thought to be most compatible with
incumbency in the sick role according to Parsons' conceptualization. The incidence of acute illnesses reported in the HIS is
substantially less for the farm population than for the other
categories (Table 2.3). The incidence for the nonmetropolitan
nonfarm population is also less than for either category of the
metropolitan population, although the difference is slight.
Differences between nonmetropolitan and metropolitan categories
appear to be greatest for children. Table 2.4 lists the inci-

Table 2.3. Acute conditions per 100 persons per year, 1969-1970

Population area	Conditions per 100 persons	
	(unadjusted for age)	*(age-adjusted)*
Central city	200.6	204.1
Outside central city	210.2	207.1
Nonfarm	200.0	199.1
Farm	159.6	163.1

Source: National Center for Health Statistics, 1974.

Table 2.4. Acute conditions per 100 persons
under age 17 per year, 1969-1970

Population area	Conditions per 100 persons
Metropolitan	298.6
Central city	287.2
Outside central city	307.2
Nonmetropolitan	272.8
Nonfarm	278.8
Farm	228.4

Source: National Center for Health
Statistics, 1974.

dences of acute conditions per 100 persons under 17 years of age
per year.

The farm population, as shown in Table 2.5, has fewer disability days than any other category of the population. The nonmetropolitan nonfarm population has more disability days than the
metropolitan population outside the central city but less than the
population in the central city. This is true for restricted activities, bed disability, and work loss whether adjusted or unad-
justed for age.

For those under 17 years of age, nonmetropolitan-metropolitan
differences were greater so that neither of the nonmetropolitan
categories was as great as either of the metropolitan categories.

Table 2.5. Days of disability per person per year by place of
residence, 1969-1970

Type of disability	Place of residence			
	Central city	Outside central city	Nonfarm	Farm
	(days per person per year)			
Restricted activity				
Unadjusted for age	16.0	13.3	15.2	12.6
Age-adjusted	15.7	13.7	15.1	11.8
Bed disability				
Unadjusted for age	7.0	5.4	6.2	4.5
Age-adjusted	6.9	5.6	6.1	4.3
Work loss				
Unadjusted for age	5.9	4.9	5.2	4.7
Age-adjusted	5.9	4.9	5.2	4.2

Source: National Center for Health Statistics, 1979.
Note: Days of restricted activity and bed disability are
adjusted to the age and residence distributions of the civilian,
noninstitutionalized population of the United States. Days lost
from work are adjusted to the age and residence distribution of
the currently employed population of the United States.

Table 2.6. Days of disability per year per person under 17
            years of age, 1969-1970

Population area	Restricted activity	Bed disability
	(days per year per person under 17)	
Metropolitan	10.2	4.8
Central city	10.5	5.2
Outside central city	10.0	4.5
Nonmetropolitan	8.6	4.0
Nonfarm	8.9	4.2
Farm	6.2	2.6

Source: National Center for Health Statistics, 1974

The differences between farm and metropolitan populations were
quite large, as Table 2.6 indicates.

Data for acute illness and restricted activities, then, indicate that the nonmetropolitan farm population uses the sick role
least while the nonmetropolitan nonfarm population occupies a position between the metropolitan populations outside and inside
central cities. For children and youth (under 17) the difference
between nonmetropolitan and metropolitan populations increases and
both categories of nonmetropolitan populations are lower than
either category of metropolitan population. It is of interest
that for the segment of population (children and youth) most dependent on the judgment of others, use of the sick role is notably
lower in the nonmetropolitan categories.

Rural and Urban Health Status

The ultimate answer to the question raised at the beginning
of this section--are rural or urban people healthier?--should lie
in comparative mortality figures. When adjusted for age, Herbert
Sauer (1976) reports that death rates of the population of nonmetropolitan counties are virtually the same as those of the
United States as a whole from 1969 to 1971. Although rural/urban
comparisons of deaths seem straightforward, in a mobile society
many people experience a combination of both rural and urban life.

Infant mortality is often used as an index of the health
status of a population. On this index, metropolitan areas have
fewer infant deaths and nonmetropolitan areas have more than the
U.S. average (Table 2.8). The differences are not large and evidence indicates that the rates are becoming more similar, showing
little difference at the present time (Mynko, 1974).

In an effort to more accurately answer the question of comparative health, Herbert Sauer calculated death rates for white
males age 35 to 74, age-adjusted by 10-year age groups using a
standard population. To minimize chance fluctuations, an 11-year
period (1959-1969) was used and data were presented by Standard
Economic Areas (SEAs) rather than by counties. SEAs were classified as either metropolitan SEAs or nonmetropolitan SEAs. Metropolitan SEAs are either similar or identical to Standard Metropolitan Statistical Areas (SMSAs) with a few exceptions and consist of one or more metropolitan counties. Nonmetropolitan SEAs
usually consist of about 6 to 20 contiguous counties that are

Table 2.7. Selected health characteristics by place of residence, United States, 1969-1970

Characteristic	All areas	SMSA					Outside SMSA		
		Total	Central city	Outside central city	Large SMSA	Other SMSA	Total	Non-farm	Farm
Percent of population with limitation of activity	11.7	10.9	11.9	10.1	11.0	10.8	13.1	13.0	13.9
Restricted activity days per person per year	14.7	14.5	16.0	13.3	14.8	14.3	14.9	15.2	12.6
Days of disability per person per year	6.1	6.2	7.0	5.4	6.2	6.1	6.0	6.2	4.5
Work-loss days per working person over 17 per year	5.3	5.3	5.9	4.9	5.3	5.3	5.1	5.2	4.7
Persons injured per 100 persons per year	26.3	26.0	24.7	27.0	27.3	25.2	27.0	27.7	22.1
Acute conditions per 100 persons per year	202.1	205.8	200.6	210.2	213.3	201.1	195.1	200.0	159.6
Short-stay hospital discharges per 100 persons per year	131.0	125.7	131.9	120.6	118.0	130.5	141.0	145.4	108.7
Surgical treatment for discharges per 1,000 persons per year (including deliveries)	70.1	72.2	73.9	70.7	69.1	74.0	66.2	68.3	60.0
Physician visits per person per year	4.4	4.6	4.7	4.5	4.9	4.4	4.1	4.3	3.2
Dental visits per person per year	1.5	1.7	1.6	1.8	2.0	1.5	1.2	1.2	1.1
Percent of population with 1+ physician visits in a year	70.7	71.8	70.6	72.8	73.1	71.0	68.5	69.4	62.4
Percent of population with 1+ dental visits in a year	45.9	48.2	44.1	51.5	50.5	46.7	41.6	41.6	41.5

Source: National Center for Health Statistics, 1974.

Table 2.8. Infant mortality rates by
            residence, 1969-1973

Residence	Infant mortality rate (per 1,000 live births)
Metropolitan	18.8
Greater	18.8
Core	19.8
Fringe	16.2
Medium	18.5
Lesser	19.4
Nonmetropolitan	20.7
Urbanized	
Adjacent	19.3
Nonadjacent	20.5
Less urbanized	
Adjacent	21.0
Nonadjacent	21.6
Totally rural	
Adjacent	21.2
Nonadjacent	21.0
U.S. total	19.3

Source: Ahearn, 1979.
Note: The original data came from the
USDHEW, 1976a.

relatively homogeneous in occupational and related activities.
There are 206 metropolitan SEAs and 303 nonmetropolitan SEAs for a
total of 509 (Sauer, 1976). Sauer compared the 25 SEAs having the
lowest death rate with the 25 having the highest (Fig. 2.2).
Twenty-two of the SEAs with the lowest death rates were nonmetropolitan. The 3 metropolitan SEAs with low death rates were relatively small areas in western states (Boulder and Colorado Springs,
Colorado: Eugene, Oregon). Twenty of the 25 SEAs with the lowest
death rates were contiguous to each other, stretching from west
central Wisconsin to Colorado, including areas in Minnesota, North
and South Dakota, Iowa, Nebraska, and Kansas. The only lowest SEA
in the South was in nonmetropolitan Arkansas. In contrast, SEAs
with the highest death rates were more evenly divided between
nonmetropolitan and metropolitan areas, although a majority were
metropolitan (11 and 14 respectively). All were located east of
the Mississippi River and concentrated in the Southeast. These
data give no credence to the contention that the health of nonmetropolitan areas is poorer than that of metropolitan areas.

    An attempt has been made by researchers at the U.S. Depart-
ment of Agriculture to construct an Index of Health Status based
on three mortality indicators (infant, total, and influenza and
pneumonia). The index was computed for each county and the indexes
for metropolitan and nonmetropolitan are averages of county indexes
for those respective categories. The U.S. index was set at 100.
On the basis of these allocations, the health status index for
metropolitan counties was more favorable (106.1) than nonmetropolitan counties (98.5). The data were displayed on a map of the
United States, with the quintile for each county shown. Counties

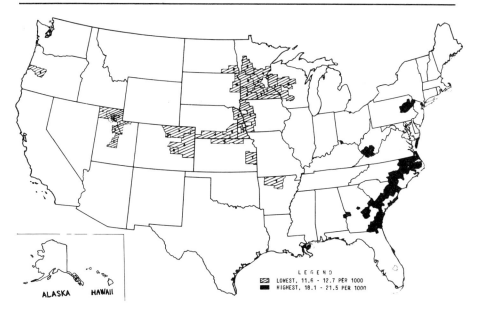

Figure 2.2.   All-causes death rates for white males age 35-74,
              25 lowest and 25 highest SEAs, 1959-1969.
              (Sauer, 1976)

in the center of the country, especially in the north central
section, show up most favorably. Much of this area is nonmetropolitan.   The South, areas of the Northeast, and the Southwest,
again much of it nonmetropolitan, show up least favorably on the
index.   The mapping shows clearly that a great diversity exists
in the health status indexes of nonmetropolitan counties.   The
comparison of index scores of metropolitan and nonmetropolitan
counties (as well as other subcategories) needs to be interpreted
with caution, however.   This is because the score for each county
is given equal weight, thus contributing equally to the index
score regardless of the size of its population.   By averaging
county index scores, the score of a county such as Kings County,
New York, with as large a population as almost one-half of the
states (2,602,012 in 1970) and a relatively low Health Status
Index (78.7), is considered equal in the calculations to the score
of Bennett County, South Dakota, with 3,088 people and a similar
Health Status Index score (76.4).   To put it another way, the low
score of Kings County, New York, is no more detrimental to the
metropolitan index than the low score of Bennett County, South
Dakota, is to the nonmetropolitan index, even though the former
has more than 800 times the population of the latter (Ross et al.,
1979).
      The general conclusion from examining mortality data is that
nonmetropolitan and metropolitan rates are similar.   Within the
nonmetropolitan population (as well as the metropolitan population)

there is a great deal of variation, so some nonmetropolitan areas
are among the healthiest places in the nation while other nonmetropolitan areas are among the least healthy. As we continue our
discussion, it should be recognized that there is no necessary
correspondence between incumbency in the sick role and age-adjusted
mortality data. One of the outcomes of greater longevity, for
example, is increased risk of chronic ailments. In this sense,
better health (using mortality as the criterion) would lead to
greater incumbency in the sick role. But in the broader sense,
incumbency in the sick role is to a considerable extent a matter
of choice that is related not only to symptoms of disease but
also to social circumstances, including society's definitions of
sickness and assessments of significant others at specific times.

Primary Groups and Social Networks Related to Use of Health Services

RURAL/URBAN DIFFERENCE IN USE OF HEALTH SERVICES

One of the most consistent findings in the utilization of health services is that rural and/or nonmetropolitan people have fewer physician calls per year than urban and/or metropolitan people. The difference is based on data from the National Health Survey (Fig. 3.1, Table 3.1). Differences are greatest in the younger ages; at the oldest ages they disappear or reverse the general rural/urban pattern.

An obvious explanation for the difference between rural and urban behavior, with regard to the use of physicians, is the difference in physician/population ratios between rural and urban (metropolitan and nonmetropolitan) settings. As indicated in Chapter 2, the difference is substantial, reaching five times as many physicians per 1,000 in the most metropolitan areas as in the most rural counties (Ahearn, 1979).

There is some evidence that challenges this particular cause and effect relationship. Using National Health Survey data, Kleinman and Wilson (1977) determined that differences were minimal in the use of physician services within nonmetropolitan areas between people located in Medically Underserved Areas (MUAs) and Adequately Served Areas (ASAs). There was no difference in the number of physician visits per year or in the proportion of the population with at least one visit per year. It should be noted that the criteria for delineating MUAs includes the physician/population ratio as well as the infant mortality rate, the percent of population 65 years and over, and the percent of the population below the poverty level.

The core finding in the study cited previously (that there is no difference in the use of physician services between persons in nonmetropolitan MUAs and ASAs) is supported by the findings of a study of four communities in rural Missouri (Hassinger and Hobbs, 1973). The communities were all in the same area, which had a common cultural base often identified with the Ozark region. They were chosen because they had different levels of health services, which ranged from the services of a part-time osteopathic physician

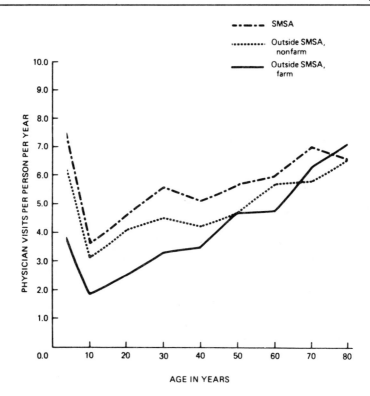

Fig. 3.1.   Number of physician visits per person per year by place
of residence.   (National Center for Health Statistics,
1979)

(the least services) to eight full-time physicians (the most).   The
latter place was the only one of the four that had hospital facilities (Table 3.2).   In Table 3.3, communities are compared by pairs
to control size and other demographic characteristics.   It was
hypothesized that differences in level of availability of services
should be reflected in differences in use of services.

The level of use of physicians (number of visits per year per
person), however, was remarkably uniform across the four communities and was not altered appreciably when age and income were controlled.   There was no evidence from this study that level of physician service within the community was a factor in level of use
of physician services.

In yet another study, Ellenbogen et al. (1959) failed to sub-
stantiate their hypothesis that different physician/population
ratios would lead to different levels of utilization in two New
York communities.

One should note that each of these comparisons is within
rural or nonmetropolitan sites.   They suggest that there is a
characteristic level of use of physicians' services in rural areas

Table 3.1. Physician visits per year, by place of residence,
            sex, and age, United States, 1975

Sex and age	All areas	SMSA	Outside SMSA Nonfarm	Farm
Both sexes				
All ages	5.1	5.3	4.6	3.8
Under 5 years	6.9	7.2	6.2	3.8
5-14 years	3.4	3.6	3.1	1.8
15-24 years	4.4	4.6	4.1	2.5
25-34 years	5.2	5.6	4.5	3.3
35-44 years	4.8	5.1	4.2	3.5
45-54 years	5.4	5.7	4.7	4.7
55-64 years	5.9	6.0	5.7	4.8
65-74 years	6.6	7.0	5.8	6.3
75 years and over	6.6	6.6	6.6	7.1
Male				
All ages	4.3	4.6	3.9	2.7
Under 5 years	7.3	7.6	6.9	4.4*
5-14 years	3.6	3.8	3.3	1.4*
15-24 years	3.3	3.6	2.8	1.5
25-34 years	3.7	4.1	2.7	1.7*
35-44 years	3.4	3.6	3.2	2.7
45-54 years	4.2	4.4	4.0	2.6
55-64 years	5.3	5.4	5.4	3.9
65-74 years	6.3	7.2	4.9	5.1
75 years and over	6.5	6.8	6.0	5.5*
Female				
All ages	5.7	6.0	5.3	4.8
Under 5 years	6.4	6.9	5.5	3.2*
5-14 years	3.2	3.3	2.9	2.2
15-24 years	5.5	5.6	5.4	3.8
25-34 years	6.7	6.9	6.2	5.0
35-44 years	6.1	6.5	5.1	4.3
45-54 years	6.5	6.9	5.4	6.7
55-64 years	6.4	6.6	6.0	5.7
65-74 years	6.8	7.0	6.4	7.7
75 years and over	6.7	6.5	7.0	9.0

Source: National Center for Health Statistics, 1979.
*Figure does not meet standards of reliability or
precision (more than 30 percent relative standard error).

Table 3.2. Professional health service characteristics of communities

Service	Pair 1 A	Pair 1 B	Pair 2 C	Pair 2 D
Number of medical doctors under 70 years of age	None	1	1	6
Number of medical doctors 70 years or older	None	None	1	None
Number of osteopaths	1/2*	1	2	2
Number of chiropractors	None	None	2	2
Hospital beds	None	None	None	42
Distance from "Metropolitan Community" (miles)	110	93	60	107
Distance from Community D (miles)	37	42	47	...
Population of center, 1960	420	266	3,176	5,836

Source: Hassinger and Hobbs, 1973, p. 514. (Reprinted by
permission of J. B. Lippincott)
*Divides time between Community A and a neighboring town.

Table 3.3. Number of visits to physician during year in four
            rural communities

Number of physician visits	Community			
	Pair 1		Pair 2	
	A (N:460) Percent	B (N:515) Percent	C (N:850) Percent	D (N:1,001) Percent
None	38.0	38.6	35.9	35.0
1-2	25.9	26.2	26.9	27.0
3-5	14.8	14.8	14.8	17.4
6-9	8.5	7.8	7.2	9.3
10 and over	12.8	12.6	15.2	11.4

Chi-square value	d.f.	Sig. level*
1) X^2 for (A)(B):0.19	4	n.s.
2) X^2 for (C)(D):9.46	4	n.s.
3) X^2 for (A)(B)(C)(D):12.50	12	n.s.

Source: Hassinger and Hobbs, 1973, p. 515. (Reprinted by
permission of J. B. Lippincott)
        *At 5 percent level.

which is little affected by differences in availability of services among rural areas. If differences in services available
among rural areas do not affect the amount of service used, it is
questionable to assume that differences in amount of service used
in rural and urban areas can be accounted for by differences of
services available (physician/population ratios) in rural and
urban areas. This interpretation is buttressed by findings that
few rural residents report being unable to obtain care when needed
(Hassinger and McNamara, 1973).

        This argument cannot be carried too far. One can conceive of
situations in which the availability of physicians would be so low
and mobility of the population so limited that use of services
would be severely reduced. That, however, is not the character of
most rural populations in the United States. Even most low-serv-
ice areas are not without physicians, and their deficiency is
mainly of specialists. Furthermore, in many of those very areas,
the populations have developed regular and effective means for
obtaining services outside the immediate community.

A SOCIOLOGICAL EXPLANATION FOR RURAL/URBAN DIFFERENCES IN
UTILIZATION OF HEALTH SERVICES
        Culture and group processes are salient variables for a
sociological explanation of rural/urban differences in physician
use. Eliot Freidson has developed a typology that intersects
elements of these variables and seems to be appropriate to the
present problem (Freidson, 1970). The congruence of lay and professional culture is one axis; the cohesiveness and extensiveness
of a lay referral network is the other. This intersection, as
shown in Table 3.4, yields the four types of health behavior described by Freidson (1970).

Table 3.4. Typology of congruence of lay and professional culture
            and strength of the lay referral structure

	Lay culture	
	Congruent with	Incongruent with
Lay referral structure	professional	professional
Loose, truncated	Type 3	Type 2
Cohesive, extended	Type 4	Type 1

        Source: Freidson, 1970, p. 294. (Reprinted by permission of
Harper & Row)

[Type 1] First, there is a system in which prospective
clients participate primarily in an indigenous lay culture
that is markedly different from that of professionals and in
which there is a highly extended, cohesive lay referral
structure. . . . In this situation the folk or indigenous
practitioner will be used by most people, and professional
practitioners will be used by few--perhaps by only the
socially isolated deviant or the desperate man clutching at
straws after all conventional devices failed.
[Type 2] The second type of lay referral system has the same
indigenous culture as the first but varies in having a truncated referral structure which allows the individual to act
entirely on his own or at least to consult no one outside of
his immediate family. While the culture of the system dis-
courages the individual from seeking a physician, reinforcement by an extended network of interpersonal influence, which
leaves the individual more vulnerable to influence by outsiders from the medical system is missing. All else being
equal, the individual may be expected to try professional
services sooner and under less desperate circumstances than
a person in the indigenous extended system.
[Type 3] The third type is the opposite of the indigenous
extended referral system. It is found when lay and professional cultures are very much alike and when the lay referral
structure is truncated. The prospective client is pretty
much on his own, guided more or less by his own understandings and experience, with few lay consultants to support or
discourage his search for help. Since his knowledge and
understandings are much like the physician's, he may take a
great deal of time trying to treat himself for disorders he
feels competent to handle, but nonetheless will go directly
from self-treatment to a physician. He is unlikely to use a
nonprofessional consultant unless the failure of the medical
system makes him desperate.
[Type 4] In the fourth type of lay referral systems, the
prospective patient is even less likely to use the services
of a nonmedical healer. It involves an extended and cohesive
referral structure and a culture similar to that of the professional. The acceptance of professional culture is considerably more likely to be reinforced than in the case of a
professionally oriented person who participates in a trun-

cated structure, and utilization of professional services is thus likely to be maximal.

In the following table Freidson's prediction of utilization of health services is explicit. Not all empirical studies support these specific predictions; notably, some have found utilization reduced or delayed where professional and lay cultures were congruent and the lay referral network was strong. This, however, does not negate the usefulness of the typology in addressing the question, and plausible alternative explanations within the framework are possible.

Table 3.5. Predicted rates of utilization of professional services, by variation in lay referral system

| | Lay culture | |
Lay referral structure	Congruent with professional	Incongruent with professional
Loose, truncated	Medium to high utilization	Medium to low utilization
Cohesive, extended	Highest utilization	Lowest utilization

Source: Freidson, 1970, p. 294. (Reprinted by permission of

The value of the typology is that it introduces social-cultural concepts as predictors of health behavior. It permits--demands--that more careful attention be given to the beliefs of people and their specific organizational structures. In the following sections the typology is used as a means of understanding the discrepancy in utilization of health services (specifically physicians' services) between rural and urban populations. It leads first to a consideration of culture (beliefs and values), followed by a consideration of primary groups and primary group networks.

The Cultural Axis
A key to the congruence of lay and professional cultures is the lay public's acceptance of the legitimacy and authority of (in this case) the medical profession. Self-medication in itself is not a rejection of the professional medical culture. In many cases, the person who self-medicates anticipates what the doctor would do if she/he were there. Advertisements for over-the-counter medications frequently use physician authority, stated or implied. Nor is the occasional use of a chiropractor or an indigenous practitioner necessarily a rejection of the authority of the regular medical profession. Only if the person adopts an opposing philosophy of health and healing and uses an alternative delivery system would his/her culture be incongruent with that of the medical profession. An example that readily comes to mind is the Christian Science adherent who rejects the authority of the medical profession and uses an alternative philosophy and mechanism of health care.
It is tempting to postulate some form of folk-scientific typology of health beliefs and practice with the expectation that

the rural sector would be closer than the urban sector to folk medicine. Lyle Saunders points out that folk medicine differs from scientific medicine in a number of ways: it is the common possession of the group; there is relatively little division of knowledge among adults; the beliefs are rooted in tradition and seem a part of the natural order; it is integrated into other elements of the culture and is reinforced by them. He observes, "Folk medicine, like scientific medicine, undoubtedly derives much of its prestige and authority from the fact that the majority of sick persons get well regardless of what is done" (Saunders, 1954).

We might expect to find traditional (as distinct from scientific) forms of healing practiced among ethnic groups such as Mexican-Americans, Native Americans, Afro-Americans, or people in areas of relative isolation such as Appalachia or the Ozarks.

Jerry Weaver (1973), for one, is critical of assigning health behavior of contemporary Mexican-Americans to a particular culture that fosters traditional healing practices. Without doubt there is traditional healing among Mexican-Americans. The *curandero* is a reality, and the beliefs associated with "hot" and "cold" substances and their relationship to health and illness are documented by Margaret Clark (1959) and others. Weaver, however, critically reviews the work that has been done on Mexican-American health behavior beginning with Lyle Saunders (1954), who emphasized the difference between Mexican-American and Anglo health cultures in the context of folk medicine. Weaver then identified second generation researchers such as Margaret Clark (1959), Arthur Rubel (1966), and William Madsen (1964) as following the lead of Saunders. They tended to regard the Mexican-American population as an undifferentiated, homogeneous mass that distrusts scientific medicine, seeks treatment from folk healers, views illness fatalistically, and sees much illness as resulting from and only curable by magic and witchcraft (Weaver, 1973). Weaver challenges this stereotypic characterization, saying that third generation research raises serious questions about the homogeneity of Mexican-American culture and of the health behavior associated with it. As evidence, in a sample from Orange County, California, Weaver found that Mexican-Americans and Anglos expressed approximately the same level of preference for receiving health care from private physicians and hospitals; and Mexican-American and Anglo parents responded similarly to the question of whether or not children should receive regular checkups. On the basis of his review, Weaver concludes that the sweeping generalizations about Mexican-American health behavior and attitudes are suspect and that the oft-claimed significance of traditional health culture is overdrawn.

A study by Harriet Kupferer (1962) of the Cherokee in North Carolina can be interpreted similarly. She divided the Native American sample into four categories according to the degree of acculturation to middle-class American society. Only those in the most conservative category were likely to utilize native medicine men, while those in the most acculturated category never did. Thus among Native Americans on a rural reservation, reliance on

folk medicine cannot be assumed. In fact, the professional practitioners were the predominant source of medical care.

The Ozarks of Missouri, it would seem, is a likely place to
find folk medicine and indigenous practitioners. A study of health
behavior in rural Missouri, while noting wide-spread use of home
medication and self-diagnosis, did not discover a lay belief system that rejects professional medical culture. In one Ozark
county, 94 percent of the respondents expressed a favorable atti-
tude toward physicians that was almost identical (95 percent) with
respondents in another rural Missouri county outside the Ozark
region (Hassinger and McNamara, 1973).

It has been suggested that the acceptance and use of marginal
practitioners such as chiropractors is an index of the extent to
which the lay culture is incongruent with the culture of professional medicine. McCorkle, for example, points out that chiropractors represent the major alternative philosophy of treatment
in the United States and suggests that the Midwest rural culture
is especially conducive to chiropractic practice (McCorkle, 1961).
In a study of the health situation in the southern Appalachian
area, however, Horace Hamilton (1962) reported a low proportion
of respondents thought that "around here people depend on chiropractors 'a great deal'" (9.5 percent) and faith healers (2 percent). He concluded: "Although these data provide only indirect
evidence of objective facts, it may be inferred that the norms and
values of modern medical science have largely replaced whatever
superstitious and unscientific ideas may have existed in the older
generation."

Moreover, the use of chiropractors is not necessarily a
rejection of mainstream medicine. While it is true that the healing philosophies of the two professions differ, this does not
necessarily mean that the layman who uses a chiropractor does so
under different assumptions than when using medical doctors. The
chiropractor, in fact, works in a cultural context of office,
equipment, and manner very similar to that of the solo medical
practitioner (Roebuck and Cowie, 1975). It was found in a study
of four rural Missouri communities that use of chiropractors was
not negatively related to education and income variables. More
important to the question being considered, the use of chiropractors was not viewed as an alternative to the use of medical doctors. Instead, chiropractors were regarded as limited practitioners who were "good for some things" and were used selectively on
that basis (Hassinger et al., 1971). The use of chiropractors is
not a good indication of rejection of professional medicine.

A key to understanding rural/urban differences in accepting
mainstream medicine may be the establishment of a family/doctor
relationship. The existence of such a relationship is evidence
that the decision makers in the family value medical care and desire access to the health care system. Consistently a high proportion of rural families in different regions of the country and
in national samples report that they have established a family

doctor relationship. Rural and urban families overall appear very
similar in the proportions reporting a relationship with a family
doctor.
    The general conclusion is that rural people are committed to
professional medicine. It is presumed, without close examination,
that urban people have a similar view. Although home treatment
and folk practices remain in urban populations as well as rural,
it is supposed that, like rural people, urban people do not base
these practices on an alternate explanation of health and healing.
The outcome of this reasoning is that the difference in beliefs
between rural and urban populations is unlikely to account for the
lower utilization of physician services in rural areas since they
are both congruent with professional health culture. Therefore,
we turn to the other axis of Freidson's model, the organizational
dimension represented by the lay referral network.

The Informal Group and Social Network Axis
    Informal groups are the woof and warp in the fabric of
community life. They are instruments of socialization, communication, and social control. The family is a particularly important
agent of socialization; through it culture is transmitted from one
generation to the next. In the family, children learn language
skills and norms of behavior. Families are also units of social
control that enforce community-approved behavior. Family relationships extend beyond the boundaries of the nuclear family to kinship
networks.
    Outside the family, much of the informal interaction takes
place in cliques--small groups based on acquaintanceship and
friendship. Typical meeting places for cliques are the street
corner, tavern, feed store, cafe, etc. Informal groups of this
type are by no means uniquely rural. In his analysis of a low-
income neighborhood in Chicago, Gerald Suttles (1968) found that
its most striking aspect was its street life, where peers of the
same sex shared the same location. Sex-exclusive peer groups were
also observed by Elliot Liebow (1967) among young black men who
hung out on Tally's Corner in Washington, D.C., and by William
Whyte (1943) in his earlier study of Street Corner Society in Boston. If anything, however, cliques are more important in rural
communities; Jack Weller (1965) reported that for men of Appalachia sex-exclusive cliques were the principal reference groups outside the family. James West (1945) found a similar situation in a
small Ozark community where major activity and conversation focused on hunting and fishing.
    Members of cliques exchange and interpret information, often
by bantering or using insider conversation. Since they are inter-
connected by overlapping membership, cliques form intricate communication networks or grapevines through which news travels.
    Informal groups are also mechanisms of social control. Infor-
mation is exchanged with approval or disapproval and sanctions are
exercised through such means as gossip and ostracism. The power of

such sanctions depends on the character of the group. For example,
among the Amish, shunning is an extremely severe sanction and a
personally devastating one.

Family, friends, and neighbors are also sources of support in
times of trouble and crisis. Illness and death are responded to in
small communities with emotional support by family and friends.
There tends to be a certain amount of looking after the elderly and
destitute (Vidich and Bensman, 1958). In this sense, the informal
bonds of the community represent a kind of social insurance for its
members.

We gain a deeper impression of the effects of informal bonds
in times of crisis when such bonds have been ruptured. Such an
event laid bare the workings of a West Virginia community when in
1972 a coal mining company dam burst, dumping 132 million gallons
of water and coal waste on residents of the Buffalo Creek area.
The area's 16 small towns were devastated. Over 125 people were
killed and 4,000 were left homeless.

The social and psychological damage, however, appeared to be
greater than the physical damage. Of the survivors examined by
psychiatrists one and one-half years after the event, 93 percent
were found to be suffering from identifiable emotional disturb-
ances. Kai Erikson (1976) says their condition could most nearly
be expressed in everyday English as confusion, despair, and hope-
lessness. "Two years after the flood Buffalo Creek was almost as
desolate as it had been the day following--the grief as intense,
the fear as strong, the anxiety as sharp, the despair as dark."
This was puzzling, because after this length of time, one would
expect the social and psychological wounds to heal.

Erikson argues that the trauma of Buffalo Creek resulted from
the disruption of the community's informal bonds, which were never
repaired. Some families left the area, others moved to higher
ground, and many found housing in government-provided house trail-
ers placed in close proximity to each other. But these were only
the outward signs of a much more basic disruption in life patterns
that resulted in a moral crisis. Erikson noted that the close
interpersonal communal ties in Buffalo Creek before the flood
seemed to be part of the natural order of things; residents were
no more aware of them than fish are of the water they swim in.
"It is a quiet set of understandings that become absorbed into
the atmosphere and thus part of the natural order" (Erikson, 1976).
When the protection of the informal bonds was torn away at Buffalo
Creek many of the people lacked the personal resources needed for
adjustment.

Here is a key to understanding the relationship between culture, group process, and behavior. The effect of subculture is
placed in the context of primary group relations. In a thoughtful
discussion, Gary Fine and Sherryl Kleinman (1979) develop the
interactionist approach by locating culture in interacting groups
and examining its diffusion through interaction among members of
the groups. Instead of variations of generalized cultural themes
or values of the larger society, subcultures are viewed as the

values, norms, and artifacts (the cultural material) of groups
that may disseminate through the society by various means. The
authors say that they conceive of a subculture

> as a set of understandings, behaviors, and artifacts used by
> particular groups and diffused through interlocking group
> networks. Such a conception (1) explains how cultural ele-
> ments can be widespread in a population, (2) explains the
> existence of local variations in cultural context through
> interactional negotiation in group settings, and (3) allows
> for an understanding of the dynamics of subcultural change.

In this context the cultural material is not a "free-floating"
mass but an integral part of the primary group process, which
includes not only the nurturing and dissemination of values and
norms but also mechanisms of social control and social support.

Relationship of Informal Groups and Social Networks to Health Behavior

With the foregoing providing a conceptual framework, attention is turned to the relationship of informal groups to health
status and the use of health services. Primary groups in the form
of families (and kinship networks), cliques, and neighborhoods
perform four functions in matters of health.

Conduits of the health culture. Through these groups, members are
socialized into the health attitudes and behaviors of the groups.
They learn definitions of health and illness, routines for meeting
problems of illness, and conditions for assuming the sick role.

Instruments of social control in health behavior. Informal groups
may require or deny members entrance to the sick-role status.
Thus parents may judge the illness of a child to be malingering
and friends and neighbors may pressure a person to obtain professional service. "How the individual's lay consultants react to
his symptoms and their acceptance of any interference with his
social functioning will do much to determine the individual's
ability to enter the sick role. The sick person will seek confirmation, advice, reassurance, and finally a form of 'provisional
validation' which temporarily excuses him from his normal obligations and activities" (Suchman, 1965).
In informal networks, judgments are made about competency and
other characteristics of health practitioners and facilities.
Thus local reputations of health services are gained through interpersonal networks.

Sources of social support in illness. Primary groups are reposi-
tories of much knowledge and skill in meeting health problems.
They provide care for which a person might otherwise seek professional help. They offer emotional support in periods of crisis,
particularly in times of illness. They offer the material means

for obtaining professional health services (for example, providing transportation to health facilities).

Channels of communication about health matters. Finally, primary group networks may serve as channels of communication in the community. Communicators of health information can take advantage of the interpersonal network in disseminating information (Ianni et al., 1960).

The Family in Health Behavior

To a high degree, decisions about seeking and using medical services occur in the family. In addition to the decision-making role, a very substantial proportion of the health care is provided within the home-family context by family members. By one estimate, 75 percent of the health care is provided without professional interventions, largely in the family context (Levin et al., 1976). Lois Pratt points out that while families usually have routine procedures for treating colds, other ailments, and injuries judged to be too trivial to warrant professional care, home medications are not limited to a narrow range of common ailments. She notes, "Over-the-counter preparations are used to treat a wide range of body systems, including the central nervous, respiratory, gastrointestinal, genital-urinary and skin" (Pratt, 1976).

Even when under professional treatment, a considerable amount of participation by family members occurs. Noncompliance or alteration in the use of prescriptions, although labeled as patient error by physicians, often is the result of conscious decisions by patients or their families based on their judgment of the progress of an illness. Pratt (1976) says, "The clearest cases of self-medication with prescription drugs occur when persons instruct physicians to provide them with prescriptions for medications, because the physicians are regarded as gatekeepers whose permission must be sought in order to carry out the desired self-medication."

Furthermore, the home is the common site of care most of the time for most chronic illnesses. Noting that only about 4 percent of those who report that they limit their activities because of chronic disease or impairment reside in institutions, Pratt (1976) points out that general hospitals treat chronically ill patients only for acute episodes and for important complications. In the case of diabetes, for example, a patient may receive perhaps 12 hours a year of medical care from doctors and nurses and the rest from family and self. "Diabetics must, in effect, become their own doctors, continually evaluating body needs, regulating food intake and injecting insulin."

Prevention and health maintenance activities are also family centered. Aside from immunization, most efforts at preventing illness and maintaining good health are left up to the individual in the family setting. Style-of-life now is recognized as a major contributor to the health of the individual. Much attention is focused on such areas as nutrition, obesity, smoking, alcoholism,

and drug abuse. And some positive health effects have been attributed to changes in life style, for example, improvement in mortality from heart disease.

It is pertinent in discussing the role of the family in
health care to note that much space in the home is devoted to
health maintenance and illness care. The bathroom is usually the
site of a medicine chest that contains prescription drugs as well
as over-the-counter medicines. Pratt (1976) describes the bathroom as being highly specialized, with body hygiene and excretion
the focal activities.

> Home bathrooms serve as shrines for carrying out elabo-
> rate health and hygiene rituals. The major ritual functions
> are: elimination, including measures to induce it; oral hy-
> giene, including cleaning teeth and dentures, medicating the
> mouth, and using dental floss or water piks; sexual hygiene,
> such as douching and applying contraceptives and menstrual
> supplies; general bodily cleansing, using soap and water or
> lotions and creams; grooming activities, such as combing and
> brushing the hair, shaving body hair, applying deodorants,
> manicuring, pedicuring, removing calluses, and applying make-
> up. Certain sicknesses such as vomiting and diarrhea are apt
> to take place in the bathroom. Most forms of home medical
> care take place there also: taking medicines; cleansing and
> applying medication and bandages to wounds; treating rashes,
> sunburn, and skin blemishes; using hot and cold water soaks;
> and removing foreign particles from various parts of the
> body. Finally, evaluations of the state of health are made
> in the bathroom: weighing the body, taking the temperature,
> and inspecting the skin, teeth and other body areas. The
> hygiene rituals tend to be carried on with a high degree of
> ceremony, and involve a vast collection of potions and para-
> phernalia that is kept in readiness in the bathroom.

Other areas of the home are associated with health and illness,
especially the kitchen in feeding the family and the bedroom when
caring for the ill at home. In the latter case, the room may be
modified and specialized equipment introduced.

In addition to the direct care provided by the family in illness, the family is the starting place for decisions to seek outside assistance in illness situations and thus likely to be the
initial step in the lay referral network that may or may not lead
to professional services. In studies of decision making in health
and illness matters, the most common interpersonal transactions
were with spouses, followed by other kin (Booth and Babchuk, 1972).

Studies of open-country residents in two Missouri counties
provide evidence of the importance of the family in maintaining
health, caring for the ill, and making decisions about entering
the health care system. In most cases an illness had to persist
over a period of time and exhibit certain signs of seriousness
before physicians were consulted. A fever was the most common

sign in alerting people to see a doctor; both the level and persistence were taken into account. A common response to the question, "At what point in an illness would a physician be consulted?"
was that the respondent (female household head) could tell when a
family member was sick enough to consult a physician. This was
most common in younger families and often involved children. It
assumed that experience with children and their ailments made it
possible to tell when children were really sick. On the basis of
these studies of rural counties it was concluded that a considerable amount of diagnosis and care commonly takes place in the
home before a physician is consulted and that each family develops
a pattern for consulting a physician (Hassinger and McNamara,
1959). Similarly, in a study of health care behavior among mothers
of a rural county in the South, it was found that common sense,
prior experience with the child, and advice from family members
were listed by an overwhelming majority of mothers as important
factors in caring for children (Peters and Chase, 1967).

Lois Pratt has related the structure of the family to personal
health practices, use of professional services, and health status.
She developed the concept of the "energized family," which has the
internal characteristics of low aversive control, low obstructive
conflict, high autonomy of members, high interpersonal support and
encouragement, and high interaction among members. A highly energized family also has multiple and dynamic ties with the broader
community. "This includes membership, leadership, and active participation by all family members in clubs, organizations and community groups; extensive use of society's varied resources; and
exposure through travel to alternative ways of life, activities,
and resources" (Pratt, 1976). The analysis developed depends on
the degree to which families meet the criteria of an energized
family and does not offer an alternative family type. However,
the traditional family with an overlay of patriarchal authority
and firm sex role prescriptions would rank low on the energized
family indexes. The considerable analysis conducted by Pratt
found that the energized pattern provides the family advantages
over the traditional family in obtaining professional health
services; the most important component of the energized family
structure in predicting use of professional services was linkages
with the broader community. The fully energized family, however,
is not a common type. In the sample for Pratt's study of an eastern city of about 150,000 population, only 10 percent of the families had attributes which classified them as fully energized;
another 20 to 30 percent were semienergized. Although not confined to any socioeconomic category, energized families were more
likely to be found among higher socioeconomic groups. It would
seem that rural families with a greater retention of patriarchal
authority and sharper division of sex roles might have fewer characteristics of the energized family.

Support within families may directly affect the health status
of family members. In a study of the consequences of unemployment
due to factory shutdown, it was found that "those men who had the

emotional support of their wives while unemployed for several
weeks had few illness symptoms, low cholesterol levels, and did
not blame themselves for the loss of the job. Those who were *both*
unemployed and unsupported had the most disturbing health outcomes.
In this study, the support of wife and friends did not result in
finding new employment sooner, but the men who had support fared
better in other respects during the period of unemployment and
made more rapid return to normal, as indicated by measures taken
at later visits" (Kaplan et al., 1977).

The Lay Referral Network
The family is a reasonable point to begin an examination of
the lay referral system, but informal networks extend beyond the
family. Jeffrey Salloway and Patrick Dillon (1973) say that a
social network is an adaptive system by which individual members
adjust to complex environments and that "when individuals become
concerned about threats--including the possibility of illness--
they begin to seek information and support from a network of social
contacts. This network is the normal set of interactions which a
person has in his daily affairs. Such networks are seen most commonly in family interaction patterns, friendship patterns, and in
work groups, and are maintained by high rates of communication,
visiting, and mutual aid."
It seems certain that informal consultation is most likely to
take place among family members. In a study of 800 adults 45 years
of age and over in Omaha and Lincoln, Nebraska, who had used a new
health resource (usually a physician), 78 percent indicated they
used interpersonal consultation in arriving at their decision.
Kin were consulted most frequently. Among kin, one's spouse was
most likely to be an advisor, followed by an adult daughter and an
adult son (Booth and Babchuk, 1972). Shifts in patterns of advi-
sors were observed by age. Middle-aged men were relatively more
likely to seek advice from friends, while elderly men were more
likely to seek advice from family members--a change which corre-
sponds to disassociation from employment.
A focal question concerns the effect of informal social networks on the utilization of health services. Freidson (1970) regards lay referral networks as resources that should facilitate
the utilization of health services (assuming that the lay and professional cultures are compatible) and he offers some empirical
evidence to support his contention. Supportive of this interpretation were Booth and Babchuk's (1972) findings that those with
fewer interpersonal relationships were more likely to delay seeking new health services.
A number of other studies, however, indicate that location of
the individual in a cohesive lay referral network delays or reduces
use of professional health services. John McKinlay questioned 87
English working-class women with regard to use of prenatal services. The women were carefully selected for common sociocultural
characteristics, so differences could not be attributed to those
factors. Forty-eight of the women were classified as underutiliz-

ers of services and 39 as utilizers. Underutilizers were more
likely to be participants in strong primary group networks and
". . . had fused or interlocking kin and friendship networks, with
which they displayed a higher frequency of interaction than did
utilizers" (McKinlay, 1973).

Nan Lin et al. (1979) found that high social support was
related to low psychiatric symptoms. In fact, the social support
scale explained more than twice as much of the illness variance as
did the combined measures of stressful life events and the demographic variables. The authors conclude that social support may
be more important than stressful life events in influencing illness symptoms.

In a study based on a sample of 503 middle- and older-aged
persons in Windsor, Canada, Roger Battistella (1971) had expected
to find greater delay in seeking services among those socially
isolated. He reasoned that family members, neighbors, friends,
and co-workers would help individuals interpret the significance
of symptoms and encourage early initiation of a physician's care.
The data did not support the hypothesis, but rather suggested the
opposite. He offers the following ex post facto explanation:

> Isolated persons may delay less because of feelings of
> apprehension, insecurity, and helplessness, which lead them
> to seek reassurance and emotional support from physicians.
> In contrast the non-isolated may have more self-confidence
> and feel more self-reliant in interpreting the significance
> of symptoms. Relatives and friends may act to alleviate
> anxiety for individuals complaining of illness by defining
> symptoms in non-serious and commonplace terms.

Edward Suchman (1964), in a study in New York City, found
that those persons in cohesive informal groups were more likely
than those not in cohesive groups to depend on the group rather
than professional services in illness. This relationship seemed
to exist regardless of the ethnic group involved. The more cohesive the group the greater the dependency of the individual upon
it for support during illness.

The studies reviewed above strongly suggest that integration
into primary groups and support from social networks reduce conditions that would lead to assuming the sick role and seeking professional care.

The relative effects of integration in cohesive primary
groups and beliefs on health behavior is demonstrated vividly in
a study by Frank Nall and Joseph Speilberg (1967). Their data
consisted of 53 Mexican-American subjects, 27 of whom had accepted
a tuberculosis treatment regimen and 26 of whom had rejected it.
Acceptance was defined as absence of resistance to entering a
sanitarium and remaining there until medically released. Rejection was strong resistance to entering the tuberculosis sanitarium
and leaving against medical advice. The authors related two sets
of variables to these behaviors: traditional beliefs and prac-

tices and integration through primary group relationships into the Mexican-American subculture.

I. The factors considered in the first set (traditional beliefs and practices)
    A. Folk beliefs
        1. *Mal ojo* (evil eye)
        2. *Mal de susto* (illness of fright)
        3. *Empacho* (food clinging to the walls of the stomach in the form of balls)
        4. Witchcraft
    B. Belief in rituals
        1. Promise making (self-deprivation of physical comfort)
        2. Visiting shrines
        3. Offering medals and candles
        4. Offering prayers
    C. Use of *curanderos* (folk curers) and folk medicine
II. The factors considered in the second set (integration through primary group relations)
    A. Integration into the family group
        1. Marital status
        2. Presence of relatives in the neighborhood
        3. Persons sought for advice on private matters
    B. Integration into the ethnic locality group
        1. Extent to which the subject "knows" the majority of people in the neighborhood
        2. Extent of visiting with neighbors
        3. Extent of intercommunity and intracommunity mobility
    C. Language
        1. Extent Spanish is used outside the home
    D. Subjective expression of social integration
        1. Alienation as measured by Srole's anomie scale

The findings were quite clear-cut. Traditional beliefs and practices were not related to following the tuberculosis regimen, while integration into the Mexican-American subculture through primary groups was associated with rejecting the tuberculosis regimen (Nall and Speilberg, 1967).

In a more general way, Gustavo Quesada and Peter Heller (1977) argue that strong primary group relationships (in this case of families) of Mexican-Americans in Texas affect use of professional health services. They say,

> While the family provides support from discrimination and estrangement of the Anglo-American society, it also strengthens cultural barriers that keep its members from participating (except in cases of extreme illness) in the health care system as patients and as health care professionals. The tendency toward extended family relationships supports the building of close-knit communities and provides further pro-

tection from the Anglo-American society. The curandero is an integral part of this community. . . . The curandero becomes a natural extension of a non-bureaucratic and deeply personal system of mutual aid.

Strong and Weak Ties in Social Networks

The answer to whether social networks promote or constrict the use of professional health services can be further refined. A useful distinction has been made between strong and weak ties in social networks. A point to be emphasized is that weak ties represent an organization style that does not imply isolation but instead often involves many interpersonal relationships with varied "others" inside and outside of the immediate community. This has led to the interesting concept of the "strength of weak ties." Mark Granovetter (1973) makes a strong case for the efficacy of weak ties in providing bridges between groups, particularly between micro and macro groups and where social distance is great. "Those to whom we are weakly tied are more likely to move in circles different from our own and will thus have access to information different from that which we receive." The paradox according to Granovetter is that weak ties, which are often portrayed in the literature as producing alienation, are, from a different perspective, seen as indispensable to individuals' opportunities to gain wide-ranging information and varied contacts. Strong ties, on the other hand, may lead to local cohesiveness, which may limit one's relationships with those who could tap resources of the larger social system. The distinction between weak and strong social ties as delineated by Granovetter does not exactly duplicate Freidson's distinction between loose-truncated and cohesive-extended lay referral structures. Freidson's loose-truncated designation emphasized the sparsity of consultants or their absence, which is by no means the character of Granovetter's weak ties. Furthermore, Freidson's cohesive-extended designation combines characteristics of both strong ties (cohesiveness) and weak ties (extensiveness). The weak-strong tie distinction can also be connected with Lois Pratt's (1976) energized family concept. The fully energized family has many and varied contacts within and beyond the community's boundaries; thus it could be characterized as being in a system of weak ties and modeling the strength of weak ties in gaining access to health services.

The designation of weak and strong ties in interpersonal relations has been applied to health behavior in a number of instances and can be extrapolated to discussions of the relative cohesiveness of primary groups to health behavior.

Based on interviews with 120 patients and short-term patients in a community mental health center in New Haven, Connecticut, Allan Horwitz (1977) examined the effects of strong and weak social networks on obtaining psychiatric treatment. His conceptual statement is based on the extent to which persons are tied into strong informal networks of interaction. "Such networks of family and friends provide emotional and instrumental support to people and the mutually reinforcing interaction within the network may delay the use of professional help." Horwitz also suggests that incumbency in a weak social network has a predictable effect on utilizing formal psychiatric services, which is not simply the absence of the effects of strong social networks. "When persons are tied to a number of other people, who are not tied to each other, they have more channels to reach information and influences and they more easily connect to social institutions" (Horwitz, 1977). Thus weak ties should facilitate accessibility to formal psychiatric agencies.

Horwitz establishes four types based on the strength of kinship ties and the openness of friendship ties. Strong kinship ties combined with closed friendship ties constitute a strong network. Weak kinship ties combined with open friendship ties constitute a weak network. He predicted that those in strong networks would have lowest access to psychiatric services through informal referral, longest delay in seeking services, and most severe symptoms before obtaining psychiatric services. The prediction was that those in weak networks would have maximum access to psychiatric services through informal referral, shortest delay in seeking services, and least severe symptoms before obtaining psychiatric services (Horwitz, 1977).

Horwitz found support for his hypotheses. "Persons with strong support from kin but without open friendship networks are insulated from informal labels and referrals and the kin network is usually able to contain all but severe problems. . . . Persons without strong kin networks but open friendship networks fulfill all our original predictions. They are the most likely group to receive informal labels and referral and to enter treatment with least severe problems and in the shortest period of time" (Horwitz, 1977). In this analysis, Horwitz attempts to correct the preoccupation of psychiatric help-seeking studies with cultural factors at the expense of structural factors. The counter to cultural interpretation for Horwitz is social network (structure) analysis. However, his conclusion is that network structures and culture are not independent factors; networks shape the cultural attitudes and values transmitted through them. This is also a possible conclusion in the analysis by Nall and Speilberg in an earlier discussed study of a Mexican-American population and their acceptance of a tuberculosis regimen.

Jeffrey Salloway and Patrick Dillon (1973) examined the effects of weak and strong ties on the utilization of health services in a sample from an ethnically mixed (40 percent black) and economically diverse census tract in suburban Boston. The dependent variables were responses to the questions:

1. (During your last illness episode) how long did it take from the first moment that you thought you might be sick until you sought treatment?

2. When was the last time you had a general physical examination?
3. When was the last time you saw a dentist?
4. When was the last time you had your eyes examined?

While relationships were not strong, friendship networks
facilitated utilization of services, while family networks were
associated with diminished rates of utilization. The authors interpret these findings in the strong ties (family), weak ties
(friendship) manner. On the basis of their findings they specu-
late that "family networks are systems which provide advice based
upon experience and role support under circumstances of threat,
but which exact a price in delayed access to medical care. Friend
networks, in contrast, might be seen as providing more information
about currently available services and little role support, but
which do not cause delay in using medical services" (Salloway and
Dillon, 1973).
Empirical research supports the hypothesis that strong ties
tend to delay and reduce use of health services. Several possible
explanations for this are:

 • Much diagnosis and care is provided by primary groups (in
particular, the family), which reduces the need for professional
services.
 • Primary group support reduces illness symptoms. As an
example, in the study by Susan Gore (1978), unemployed workers
with strong family support had fewer illnesses than unemployed
workers without strong family support.
 • Strong social networks in their social control role serve
as validators of illness; as such, they have the power to invali-
date illness.
 • The process of consultation may reduce anxiety, which in
turn may reduce use of health services.

In general, the effect of weak social networks is not simply a
reduction in the effects of the strong social networks. The
refinement of the concept helps to understand that weak social
networks have an independent role in the use of health services,
which is captured in the idea of the "strength of weak ties"
(Granovetter, 1973). The essential idea is that weak ties provide
the individual with far-ranging and diverse contacts including
numerous contacts with professional health resources. There are
several possible explanations for this:

 • With weak ties, more consultants can be reached. Thus more
information about, and connections to, health services are available.
 • Weak ties tend to reach beyond the immediate community and
thus provide access to extralocal health resources.
 • Weak ties can bridge social distance more efficaciously

than strong ties and thus provide access to a greater range of information and resources.

APPLICATION TO RURAL AREAS OF FINDINGS ABOUT THE RELATIONSHIP OF
PRIMARY GROUP STRUCTURES AND SOCIAL NETWORKS TO HEALTH BEHAVIOR
In the previous discussion only passing reference was made to rural areas. Unfortunately the key studies with regard to effectiveness of primary groups and social networks have been conducted in urban settings. The objective of the review, however, was to gain insight into factors that account for rural/urban differences in utilization of health services.

Freidson's typology has the advantage of directing attention to the interaction of organizational (lay referral network) and cultural (beliefs and values) variables. Professional medical care is widely accepted and the physician is regarded as *the* authority in matters of health. This is true of rural populations who, by using the criterion of having a family doctor, are as firmly connected to the medical care system as are other population categories. This and other evidence suggests that the cultural side of Freidson's paradigm is not a major contributor to the rural/urban difference in use of health services. The studies did show, however, that strong primary group relationships led to delayed or reduced professional health care. Therefore, the explanation for differences in rural/urban use of health services seems to hinge on the characteristics of the primary group relationships and the social networks which they form. A very useful conceptual refinement has been made and empirically supported by distinguishing strong and weak ties in interpersonal relationships.

The Primary Group-Social Network Structure of Rural Society
An argument often advanced is that the organizational structure of rural communities is different from that of urban communities and that the difference has predictable consequences for health behavior. Rural/urban differences in organizational structure is a venerable theme based on Emile Durkheim's proposition that social differentiation increases with population density and found in Toennies' *gemeinschaft-gesellschaft* typology. Richard Dewey (1960) developed five qualities related to size and density of population.

• Anonymity--the ability to remain unknown as a person (nameless) even though one sees many people. According to Dewey, "Anonymity is inevitable for the vast majority of a city's population and impossible at the rural extreme, save for the hermit."
• Division of labor--must increase as the size and density of population increases. "Whereas small communities can present a relatively undifferentiated occupation pattern, a city of a million cannot." The extreme example is the traditional agricultural village where virtually the entire population is engaged in agri-

culture with few commercial activities. Most rural communities
are not occupationally homogeneous to that extent, but they tend
to revolve around a single occupation such as farming, mining,
fishing, lumbering, or recreation. When industry moves to rural
areas, greater division of labor occurs and the community takes on
a more urban character.

• Heterogeneity of the population--along such lines as race,
nationality, religion, social class, and life-style increases
with size and density of population. Cities of size are conglom-
erates of people of different cultural backgrounds and life-
styles. While divisions of these kinds occur in rural communities, they are less common; hence, rural people are not as tolerant of different life-styles.

• Impersonal and formally prescribed relationships--formal
rules increase with size and density of population. In large
cities, formal rules are needed; good intentions and informality
will not suffice to induce minimal order. In small communities,
social control can be maintained informally through groups using
such sanctions as gossip and ostracism.

• Symbols of status that are independent of personal ac-
quaintance--increase with size and density of population. In the
anonymity of the city, one needs impersonal symbols to identify
the status of those with whom one interacts. For example, police-
men, nurses, and waitresses wear uniforms as symbols of their status. White collars and blue collars are similar status symbols.
In rural communities, people know the status of each other without
the outward symbols. Everyone knows the town marshal and a uniform would be out of place. The millionaire farmer does not need
the symbol of dress to distinguish him from his less affluent
neighbor.

Thus, according to Dewey, urban communities are characterized
by anonymity, high division of labor, heterogeneous population,
formal rules, and impersonal symbols of status. Rural communities
are characterized by personal relationships, low division of
labor, homogeneous population, informal rules, and status based on
personal knowledge. These sets of characteristics represent end
positions on a rural-urban continuum and group processes reflect
the character of the respective settings.

Evidence of primary group support networks. Social organization on the rural side of the continuum is regarded as more primary in the sense that it is smaller, more personal, and less
specialized. Some would challenge this empirically, using the
certain evidence that primary groups are essential components of
both urban and rural communities. Secondary-type relationships
become more prevalent as rural communities enter the mainstream of
the larger society (Vidich and Bensman, 1958).

But evidence as it exists supports the orthodox view that
primary groups and social networks of strong ties are relatively
more important in rural than urban areas. Rural families are more

likely to be stable, as indexed by lower divorce rates and higher fertility rates (Beale, 1978).

The importance of interpersonal relationships in rural areas has been demonstrated by the body of work on diffusion and adoption of agricultural innovations (Lionberger, 1960; Rogers and Shoemaker, 1971). An important element in this work is the identification of social cliques and neighborhoods and tracing the flow of information through the resulting interpersonal networks. Attention is also given to the validation of proposed innovations by "friends and neighbors" as an important stage in the adoption process. The findings of this body of research support the belief that informal groups are prevalent in rural communities and important in disseminating information. The research also demonstrates the effectiveness of certain persons (influentials) in validating proposed agricultural practices. In total, the research on dissemination and adoption of agricultural innovations represents the most sustained effort in the sociological literature to understand the effects of social networks on an area of behavior.

Work by Miller and Crader (1979) in Utah indicates that rural community satisfaction is based on interpersonal relationships more than in urban communities, while satisfaction in urban communities is based more on economic factors.

Angus Campbell (1981), using national samples for research conducted at the Institute for Social Research, University of Michigan, says,

> If we order the localities within which people live from the largest metropolitan places to the most rural, we find indeed predictable differences in the way people describe their lives. It is surely true that the large cities are less sociable than the rural communities. Nearly a quarter of the white people in the metropolitan centers say they have never visited the home of any of their close neighbors; in the rural counties this figure is near 5 percent. Nearly one in ten of the white metropolitan residents do not know the name of any of their closest neighbors; in the rural areas hardly more than 1 percent. City people are less likely than rural people to feel they have a number of close friends or describe their lives as generally friendly. The sense of living among strangers clearly increases with the size of the community in which one lives.

Informality persists in institutional areas of rural society including commerce, education, religion, and government (Vidich and Bensman, 1958). Thus the rural church has many of the characteristics of a primary group of friends and neighbors; local government is conducted in an informal consensual manner rather than a formal conflictual manner.

At this point, it would be desirable to demonstrate the effects of differences in the organizational structure of rural and urban communities on the utilization of health services. Unfortunately definitive comparative data in this framework do not exist. Some support, however, is offered for the claim that rural populations depend more on primary groups and lay referral networks in health behavior than do urban populations. Susan Gore (1978) reported significantly higher social support and fewer illness symptoms among a group of unemployed rural workers than among a similar urban group. Mynko (1974) has produced the most comprehensive synthesis of the rural health literature pertaining to health status, availability of health services, perception of health and medical care, and utilization of health services. Except for the first, in each topic, she considers "non-professional" health services which include "the personnel, facilities, delivery mechanisms, and paraphernalia that seek to give rehabilitative, curative, and/or preventive medical care, but are not recognized or licensed through professional medical societies and/or boards" (Mynko, 1974). Among nonprofessional personnel are self-diagnosticians, lay practitioners, medicine men or faith healers, and untrained midwives.

Mynko finds some consensus in the various authors' conclusions about rural and urban nonprofessional care and presents these in propositional form with whatever evidence is in the literature. The position at which Mynko arrives, on the basis of her review, is that *rural persons have more locally available nonprofessional medical care than urban persons.*

Although little systematic, well-defined study has been found in this area, it seems that rural persons have more nonprofessional personnel available to them. This tendency was shown for self-diagnosticians, lay practitioners, and especially midwives. . . . Turning to the delivery methods of the nonprofessional system, it seems that rural persons have a more extensive lay referral system, lay health education system, and have organized the folk system in a division of labor that is compatible with professional medicine. Nonprofessional care seems to be most available to rural persons for chronic non-incapacitating conditions, while professional services deal with critical incapacitating conditions [Mynko, 1974].

A summary of the statement of the effect primary groups and social networks have on the utilization of services in rural and urban areas must be in hypothetical form:

• Primary groups and strong social networks are relatively more important in rural than urban areas. Therefore, the consequences that these social structures have on utilization of health services should be accentuated for rural areas.
• Primary groups and strong social networks operate as factors to reduce use of services
       - by providing alternatives to professional treatment such as home treatment,

   - by offering support that might otherwise be sought from
professional sources,
   - in the role of validators of illness, by denying the status of illness to some individuals, and
   - by delaying seeking professional services through the
process of network review.
   • Weak social networks and energized families are relatively
more important in urban than rural areas. Therefore, the consequences of these social structures should be accentuated for urban
areas.
   • These kinds of social structures contribute positively to
the utilization of professional health services
   - by providing more contacts with the professional health
care system,
   - by providing more diverse contacts with the professional
health care system, and
   - by bridging social and physical distances.

SOCIAL PRACTITIONERS' USE OF PRIMARY GROUP AND SOCIAL NETWORK
STRUCTURES
   The application of primary group and social network structures has not been lost to human services practitioners. Community workers have almost instinctively used natural groups and
social networks as they have sought to disseminate information and
initiate change. The eager acceptance by agricultural extension
agents of rural sociological research on diffusion and adoption of
agricultural innovations is explained in part by its scientific
legitimation of what extension personnel had been doing for a long
time. County agents could visualize in precise sociometric patterns the networks of people they worked with, identifying clique
boundaries and differentiating groups according to sociocultural
criteria. They could also spot "influentials" who were the focus
of a communication network on a mind's map of interpersonal relationships. The trick was to plug into the network at the right
places for efficient dissemination and validation of information.
   There is a growing awareness among practitioners that the
availability of informal support is crucial to success in preventing or delaying the institutionalization of chronically impaired
persons. Burton Dunlop (1980) concludes that the bulk of care
received by chronically impaired persons is provided informally,
principally by family members. Thus elderly persons having family
or other nonprofessional support that provided intermittent but
sustained care were able to remain out of nursing homes longer
(and until their impairments were considerably more serious) than
were elderly persons without informal support mechanisms. In an
article dealing with mental health, Roger Nooe (1980) advocates
deinstitutionalization in rural areas. He thinks that rural areas
have special characteristics that contribute to deinstitutionalization of mental patients. "Generally, these rural residents
nurture a strong sense of responsibility for others and have a

number of natural support systems which include families, churches
and civic groups."

Rural people may regard a greater range of idiosyncratic
behavior as being within a tolerable range. This judgment is
supported by the study by Elaine and John Cumming (1957), which
found that lay people in a rural Canadian community denied the
existence of mental illness in hypothetical cases with clear pa-
thologies from a professional point of view.

In a more general statement, Raymond T. Coward (1978) considered the utility of "natural helping systems" in the delivery
of rural services along with some of the pitfalls. He notes that
the study, development, and use of strong natural helping systems
is increasingly seen as a top priority for community psychologists
and practitioners interested in the delivery of human services.
In the past, these networks were seen as a major force in accounts
of the "spontaneous recovery or remission" of psychological disorders. More recently, attention has shifted toward the role such
networks can assume in preventive or crisis intervention.

In reviewing the use of natural helping networks in a remote
Alaska area, Coward points out possible pitfalls. He cites a case
in which native leaders, respected for their wisdom and experience, were recruited as public welfare aides. The effort was "designed to bridge the gap between the everyday needs of the natives
living in remote areas and the severe limits of the professional
staff to meet these needs because of distance, cultural and lin-
gual barriers, and lack of time" (Coward, 1978). Native leaders
were trained and sent back to their communities to carry out tasks
formerly performed by caseworkers. Coward faults this tactic:
"Despite the fact that they [native leaders] were chosen because
of their natural helping skills, the project proceeds to put them
through a nine-month training period where they learned the ins
and outs of public welfare--they became junior social workers."
However, because of the remoteness of the area and general neglect, "they reverted back to their more natural skills and became
actively engaged in providing practical, immediate help to their
neighbors" (Coward, 1978).

Coward insightfully concludes,

> The Alaskan Welfare project reflects the most common strategy
> for involving natural systems--one which attempts to co-opt
> the leaders of the natural system and simply make them exten-
> sions of the burgeoning human service bureaucracy. The Alas-
> kan aides were somewhat able to resist this process because
> of their remoteness from the main body of professionals;
> however, in most projects of this type the natural helpers
> end up taking their place at the bottom of the agency hier-
> archy--an act which often serves to diminish their status,
> influence and power.

Instead of coopting the natural helping networks, Coward advocates
forming new and innovative alliances with them--adapting the proj-

ect to the network's idiosyncratic style of functioning. This is
different from manipulating the helping network to fit the agency's program.

     In rural areas, institutional groups may be quite informal
and take on aspects of primary group relations. Rural churches
are a leading example; they are often the focus of a network of
communication and behavior validation. John Hatch and Jo Ann Earp
found this to be true in a predominantly black county in Mississippi. The church provided a natural social structure that was
effectively utilized in introducing a new health facility and
program into the county. Hatch and Earp report that the small
churches were primary groups where members were often related by
blood or marriage. The church was the most influential social
structure (formal or informal) outside the family in the lives of
these very poor rural people.

     As such, the church often served as a primary resource for
     intervention in family groups or kinship networks in times of
     crisis. As both the most influential institution and the
     acknowledged source and initiator of practical instructions
     on daily problems, it helped set the established code of con-
     duct for people's daily lives and enforced sanctions against
     those who violated that code. Finally it acted as the com-
     munication center for all the affairs taking place in the
     community and seemed to legitimate the aims and methods used
     by newcomers or outsiders wishing to "organize" or otherwise
     intrude in community affairs. Thus the church structure was
     an important model as well as a participator in the success-
     ful initiation and operation of any community organizational
     effort in Mound Bayou. The style and structure of the North
     Bolivar County Health Council, which later developed as the
     overall coordinating agency for the comprehensive health
     center plus other community development efforts, was closely
     patterned on the local church organization [Hatch and Earp,
     1976].

     Hatch extended this understanding of the "natural social
structure" of rural black communities to North Carolina in implementing a community health education program. Hatch and Kay
Lovelace (1980) report:

     Significant life events centering around the church, such as
     celebrations of birth, marriage, and death, continue with
     little change from earlier days. The church provides a
     setting for the exchange of news, social support, and re-
     sources. For instance, important social events in the commu-
     nity are announced at church, and after services the church
     members informally exchange various bits of information, give
     accounts of friends and family, and often arrange for ex-
     change of labor and other resources. The church continues to
     play a significant role as well in caring for the ill and

giving support to families in times of crisis. These observations led us to the notion that by building on and expanding the support role these churches were already playing--
that is, providing knowledge, advice, and other forms of help
to friends, relatives, and neighbors--the level of sound
health knowledge and the effectiveness of advice-giving could
be increased. Further, we hypothesized that the church would
afford an effective and efficient means for intervention in
certain selected health conditions that disproportionately
affect people in rural black communities.

In the health profession, there is greater recognition of the
role of indigenous persons in delivering health services. One of
the advantages of physician extenders and other auxiliary practitioners often cited is that they are likely to be drawn from the
community they serve. Physicians, especially psychiatrists, are
more likely now than formerly to recognize the value of indigenous
practitioners such as Indian medicine men or *curanderos* among
Mexican-Americans in the Southwest. In-service training of local
personnel has been a hallmark of neighborhood health centers, both
rural and urban. It not only provides employment for mostly poor
people, but also is thought to reduce social distance between
health care institutions and patients.
    Eva Salber has reported on a number of studies she has done
in rural counties of North Carolina. She believes the medical
care system should make more and better use of patients' social
networks. Salber advocates use of "health facilitators"--layper-
sons to whom others naturally turn for advice, support, and counsel. The lay referral network, according to Salber (1979), would

- strengthen the professionals' ties with the community,
- channel knowledge to and from the community,
- educate the community about the roles and functions of
medicine and the professional about the lay referral and lay consultant system.
- acquaint the community with available human service resources,
- improve the helper's role in helping others so that all who
need help are reached and strengthened,
- lessen the dependency and passivity of the patient in relation to the professional, and
- help the patient cope more effectively with his/her problem.

In the utilization of indigenous practitioners, local trainees, and health facilitators, the health care professions have
assumed that new personnel would be incorporated into the regular
health care system without changing it. This is the classic definition of cooptation offered by Philip Selznick (1953). For
example, professional medicine's interest in native practitioners
such as medicine men and *curanderos* is based on an attempt to

intellectualize the reasons for their use and to assign psychological bases for their success. Above all, toleration of these
types of practitioners does not alter the philosophical, knowledgeable, or organizational bases underlying the dominant medical
care system (Martinez, 1977). Medical sociology researchers could
be accused of contributing to the cooptation of lay networks and
indigenous practitioners. So long as they were more or less un-
recognized as major contributors to health care they were left
alone, but when they were "discovered" they became subject to manipulation by organizations of the larger society. Like tundra,
lay networks are present and absolutely essential, but also like
tundra, these networks are fragile and subject to destruction by
forces attempting to do good.

The most radical critique of the health care system is based
on damage it is purported to do. Ivan Illich (1976) devotes
attention to documenting clinical iatrogenesis--damage done by
physicians and the medical care system. But more important in the
overall scheme are social and structural iatrogeneses created by
medical bureaucracies that manipulate patients as consumers. The
outcome is addiction to the medical care system and loss of autonomy by individuals in coping with personal problems. Illich's
solution involved deprofessionalization and debureaucratization of
health services and a radical return to self-care and self-respon-
sibility.

Self-help groups (many of which deal with specific health
problems) may be an effort to regain primary group-social networks.
Alan Gartner and Frank Riessman (1977) say that their rapid pro-
liferation "not only reflects the decline of traditional integrating institutions such as the family, the church, and the
neighborhood, but it also reflects the inadequacy of formal care-
giving institutions in meeting needs that arise in the absence of
these bonding structures." They say that self-help groups derive
their power by combining a number of properties, including helper-
therapy principle, aprofessionalism, consumer intensity, use of
indigenous or peer support, and demand for individuals' participation. Gartner and Riessman (1977) recognize the problem of cooptation of self-help groups by professional agents.

> At one level, it can be argued that the self-help groups by
> their very essence are nonprofessional and that any profes-
> sional involvement might contaminate them in a variety of
> ways. They might attempt to imitate professional practice;
> they may be coopted by the professionals, or dominated by
> them; they might lose their purity, their simplicity, and
> their closeness to the people and their problems.

Self-help groups, however, may function successfully outside
the professional milieu. An example is Alcoholics Anonymous, a
lay organization that incorporates elements of primary group and
lay network support. Originally disparaged by professionals, its

subsequent success demanded recognition by the medical profession. The program, however, has resisted efforts of professionalization and cooptation.

In this extended discussion, a case has been made that primary groups and primary social networks serve in some ways as an alternative to use of professional services. To the extent that these social structures are more prevalent in rural areas, use of professional services should be lower in rural areas. Furthermore, if it can be argued that a reduction in the use of professional health services because of the mechanisms of social support is not detrimental to health status, then the lower use of professional health services in rural areas need not be seen as a problem but rather as an advantage.

Regionalization: Concept, Perimeters, and Landmarks

Regionalization, as used here, refers to the coordination of differentiated service units in a given area. Thus the principal elements of regionalization of services are differentiation of services, ordered distribution of services, and coordination of services. The concept has special relevance for rural society because of the strong tendency of rural institutions to be connected with those of the larger society and to be controlled from nonlocal sources.

Certain distinctions need to be made regarding regionalization if it is to be used in a sociological discussion of rural health. Consideration needs to be given to the sociological character of the concept (the use of regionalization has been largely in health planning rather than in sociological discourse), its relationship to other spatial concepts (regionalism, social areas, and trade areas), and its substantive connection to rural social organization.

THE SOCIOLOGICAL CHARACTER OF REGIONALIZATION

Specialization or differentiation of services is a needed condition for regionalization. A regionalized service system conforms well to Durkheim's conceptualization of organic solidarity based on a division of labor (Durkheim, 1964). This condition is fully met in modern health care systems where differentiation exists seemingly to the point of fragmentation.

The second principal element in regionalization is the patterned distribution of services. One looks to human ecology for discussions of this aspect of the concept. Amos Hawley (1950), for example, develops an analysis of the interdependence of trade centers, showing the dominant-subdominant relationships among them. In rural areas, economic and professional services are provided in trade centers located at fairly regular intervals from each other. At one time trade centers tended to be quite uniform in the services they offered clients living in their immediate hinterlands. Compatible with this patterning, physicians were widely dispersed and were likely to be found in places as small as 500 to 1,000 population. Through greater mobility associated with better transportation and the changing aspirations of rural people, the service relationships between trade centers and hinterland populations have changed. Clients today range more widely in seeking specialized services. A hierarchical pattern has emerged with different centers providing different levels of specialized services. Differentiation and interrelationships of service centers has been the subject of numerous theoretical and empirical treatments of the spatial organization of services. The landmark work of Walter Christaller (1933/1966) on central place theory has had profound influence on subsequent treatment of the spatial organization of services.

Organizationally, regionalization represents a special type of interorganizational coordination, and it is useful to place the concept in that context. Once a neglected area, research on interorganizational networks has taken significant strides in recent years. Some of the leading work in this area has been related specifically to health care organizations (Levine and White, 1961; Mott, 1968; Lehman, 1975). In interorganizational analysis, emphasis is on the interorganizational field itself. Roland Warren et al. (1974) observed in the interorganizational fields they studied that there were sets of norms which governed the range of acceptable behavior among the constituent organizations. These were grounded in a basic consensus or common "institutionalized thought structure." The authors say, "Perhaps the most important global aspect of the organizational field is this basic agreement on definition of social reality and social problems, respective agency domains, and ground rules for interaction, within which interaction is limited both in frequency and in scope of the issues involved." Groups that do not conform to the "culture of the field" are either pressured into line or excluded from participation in the network.

Regionalization of services, it should be remembered, represents a special type of interorganizational coordination. The special quality of the coordination is that the services are differentiated on the basis of specialization and spatially distributed in a hierarchical manner. Thus the organizational imperatives of division of labor that are based on specialization apply. Specifically, specialized parts need to be integrated in order to provide comprehensive services that are appropriate, available, and efficient. Failure to integrate services results in fragmentation, duplication, and inappropriate services--conditions of which the health care delivery system is often accused. Regionalization results in the centralization of more specialized services into larger service organizations. Centralization of control tends to accompany centralization of services, which is why people in the hinterland often express fear that regionalization means loss of control to centers that, while not as remote as Washington or Chicago, are nonetheless outside their immediate influence.

The issue of centralization and decentralization is quite

different when viewed from a national perspective. For the central
bureaucracies of the national society, regionalization represents
a move toward decentralization. In order for the central bureaucracies to get programs to the people, they need to have a manage-
able number of "local" contact points--organizations with which
the bureaucracies can relate (the bureaucracies simply cannot
interact with groups which do not keep records and maintain sta-
bility). The formation of regionalized delivery systems tends to
meet this need.

REGIONALIZATION RELATED TO OTHER SPATIAL CONCEPTS

Regionalism
        There are a number of other concepts with spatial elements
that need to be identified if only to distinquish them from regionalization. Perhaps most important is regionalism. In the
International Encyclopedia of the Social Sciences, regionalism is
defined as the scientific task of delimiting and analyzing regions
as entities lacking formal boundaries, with a region being "a
homogeneous area with physical and cultural characteristics distinct from those of neighboring areas. As part of a national domain a region is sufficiently unified to have a consciousness of
its customs and ideals and thus possess a sense of identity distinct from the rest of the country" (Vance, 1968). During the
1930s and 1940s major contributions were made to the regional literature by sociologists, especially those at the University of
North Carolina, by examining the South as a region. The unique
social and cultural characteristics of the South were related to
such problems as poverty and underdevelopment (Vance, 1929; Odum,
1936; Raper, 1943). A regional literature was also developed for
the Great Plains, with strong emphasis on the relationship of the
physical environment to settlement patterns and socioeconomic
development (Webb, 1936; Kraenzel, 1953). Ethnic identity may be
a key element in regional analysis, as it is in the Southwest with
its large Mexican-American population.
        A popular application of regionalism is Joel Garreau's
writing in the *Washington Post* where he suggests that instead of
50 states there are nine distinct regions (he calls them nations)
of North America, the boundaries of which do not follow state
lines and reach into Canada, Mexico, and the Caribbean islands.
Their names and capitals are: the Breadbasket, Kansas City;
Ectopia, San Francisco; the Foundry, Detroit; the Empty Quarter,
Denver; the Islands, Miami; Mex America, Los Angeles; New England,
Boston; Dixie, Atlanta; Quebec, Quebec. Garreau (1979) remarks
of the nine nations, "Each is distinct--organized by money resources, topography, music, poetry, and unique webs of history.
Most important, each nation has its own way of looking at things--
at itself and at the other eight nations."
        Thus although regionalization and regionalism share spatial
identity, they are clearly different concepts. Regionalization

represents organizational aspects of space, while regionalism de-
notes areas of sociocultural unity.

Social Areas and Trade Areas

A distinction can also be drawn between social areas and
regionalization. Social areas are usually delineated in a manner
similar to regions on the basis of homogeneity of one or more
social and/or economic indicators. The basis for social area
analysis in cities was developed by Shevky and Williams (1949)
and Shevky and Bell (1955). The original work delineated social
areas in Los Angeles on the basis of three measures: (1) social
rank, measured by occupation and education; (2) urbanization,
measured by fertility, gainfully employed women, and proportion of
single-dwelling residences; and (3) segregation, measured by eco-
logical segregation of ethnic or racial groups. Cecil Gregory
(1958) delineated rural social areas of Missouri based on homogeneity of a large number of socioeconomic indicators. Four areas
and eight subareas in the state were identified.

Another spatial concept, namely trade area (or service area),
is closer to that of regionalization. Trade area research includes Charles Galpin's (1915) work on community delineation and
Walter Christaller's (1933/1966) central place analyses. Although
developed separately, trade areas and regionalization tend to deal
with the same type of unit and some of the same organizational
problems. Therefore, insights developed in trade center research
appear to be useful when discussing the spatial aspects of regionalization.

IMPLICATIONS OF REGIONALIZATION OF HEALTH SERVICES FOR RURAL AREAS

If anything is clear about rural American society, it is that
it is enmeshed in the larger society. Local rural institutions
(governments, churches, schools, health organizations, etc.) are
linked with nonlocal (state, regional, and national) organizations
in what Roland Warren (1978) calls vertical relationships. The
outside participant in the process is often represented by the
bureaucracies of government, ecclesia, or business. A common observation is that decisions that affect local communities such as
where to build roads are often made outside the community.
Warren makes the point forcefully:

> An important characteristic of the vertical pattern is the
> rational, planned, bureaucratically structured nature of the
> extracommunity ties. . . . They are structured along bureau-
> cratic administrative lines, and the relation of the local
> unit to the extracommunity system is usually clearly pre-
> scribed in terms of the overall objectives and operating pro-
> cedures of that system. The particular form of the relation-
> ship to the larger system is not left to chance: in Sumner's
> terms not "crescive" but "enacted." Consequently, the local

community unit is an integral part of a rationally ordered, bureaucratically administered extracommunity system.

Regionalization, as it applies to health services, is a statement of the vertical linkages of a particular service system. In some ways it mirrors the expansion of the boundaries of the local community; however, the services offered beyond the secondary level are almost certain to be outside the rural community. Even more critical, the centralization of services beyond the local community also centralizes decision making and administration. In this light, regionalization is an especially intriguing concept in that it deals with the vertical relationship which is so important to understanding the modern rural community and rural society.

As regionalization becomes more important in organizing health services, it is essential to account for its effects on rural population. There are a number of issues involved, among them:

• The Urban to Rural Power Issue--Regionalization implies local centralization of services; consequently, the relative weakness of hinterland-to-center relationships is an important consideration for rural areas.

• The Consumer Issue--Many regionalization models offer remote-area services through physicians' assistants or nurse practitioners. There are questions about the acceptance of such practitioners and the quality of their services.

• The Technological Imperative--Complex and sophisticated technology needs a large and stable resource base. The center unit in regionalized organizations may monopolize resources at the expense of the outlying units.

• The Spatial Issue--As services are centralized, some persons in the hinterland may become more physically isolated than before regionalization.

• The Governance Issue--The failure of regional programs is often attributed to the lack of control of the various units. Corporate control is one solution, but corporate control may have built-in rigidity and unwanted monopolistic tendencies.

• The Political Issue--As a rational-efficiency model, regionalization comes up against political pressure groups in deciding the location of services and development of programs.

• The Domain Issue--Regionalization may tend to institutionalize the domains of units involved and prevent new elements from entering the system.

REGIONALIZATION IN HEALTH DELIVERY

Regionalization has found greater acceptance in health delivery activities than in sociological analysis. In discussing regionalization from the health planner's point of view, David Pearson (1976) says, "The term 'regional personal health services' is used to explain the process that brings consumers and providers of medical care together in a defined area with discrete facilities separated by space and hierarchical service responsibilities but functionally linked in a formal structured, and coordinated manner."

Pearson goes on to say that the joint application of the concepts of geographic and organizational regionalization provides a structure within a given boundary or geographic area for deployment of various consumer goods and services, based on the logic of regional location and developing from regional planning, decentralization, and coordination.

This sort of regionalization involves the principles of optimal allocation, distribution, and use of resources and the maximization of output, as well as the socio-economic concept of providing goods and services within defined locales. . . . The essential elements of the resulting structure are an economically, socially, and spatially defined region and an organization that combines centralization and decentralization to permit a two-way flow of activity and coordinated effort [Pearson, 1976].

Pearson's elaboration of the definition reveals the underlying advocacy of many health planners for regionalization. Essentially, regionalization is a rational-efficiency model seen as a solution to the problems of health service delivery which result from gaps and overlaps in services. Referring specifically to emergency medical services, but with broader implications, Geoffrey Gibson (1977b) says that since 1973 the major organizational theme in the United States has been regionalization of health services. He notes further that regionalization is not being merely encouraged, but is required by governmental and non-governmental agencies such as the Robert Wood Johnson Foundation as a condition for funding.

Landmarks toward Regionalization of Health Services

Dawson Report. Although regionalized health care systems were present earlier in Sweden and Denmark, the Dawson Report (The Report of the Consultative Council on Medical and Allied Services, May 1920, chaired by Lord Dawson of Penn) is credited by many as being the earliest formal regional health proposal in western society (Pearson, 1976). The Dawson Report was influential in developing the British health care system and has become a point of reference for regionalized models in the United States.

The Dawson Report discussed domiciliary services that were usually provided in the patient's home or in the consulting room of the general practitioner. Domiciliary services included those of doctor (general practitioner), dentist, pharmacist, nurse, midwife, and health visitor. The range of activity at this level was broad, with consideration being given to prevention.

23. We think that in any scheme of improved medical services the duty of the general practitioner to advise how to prevent disease and improve the conditions of life among his patients should be an important element in his work.[1]

In addition to domiciliary services, health services were perceived as being provided at three levels of health centers-- primary, secondary, and teaching hospitals (tertiary). The Dawson Report says:

9. . . . A Health Centre is an institution wherein are brought together various services, preventive and cura- tive, so as to form one organization. Health Centres may be either Primary or Secondary, the former denoting more simple, and latter a more specialized service.

10. The domiciliary service of a given district would be based on a *Primary Health Centre*--an institution equipped for services of curative and preventive medicine to be con- ducted by the general practitioners of that district, in con- junction with an efficient nursing service and with the aid of visiting consultants and specialists. Primary Health Cen- tres would vary in their size and complexity according to lo- cal needs, and as to their situation in town and country, but they would for the most part be staffed by the general prac- titioners of their district, the patients retaining the serv- ices of their own doctors.

11. A group of Primary Health Centres should in turn be based on a *Secondary Health Centre*. Here cases of diffi- culty, or cases requiring special treatment, would be re- ferred from Primary Centres, whether the latter were situated in the town itself or in the country round. The equipment of the Secondary Centres would be more extensive and the medical personnel more specialized. Patients entering a Secondary Health Centre would pass from the hands of their own doctors under the care of the medical staff of that centre. Whereas a Primary Health Centre would be mainly staffed by general practitioners, a Secondary Health Centre would be mainly staffed by consultants and specialists.

13. Secondary Health Centres should in turn be brought into relationship with a *Teaching Hospital* having a Medical School. This is desirable, first in the interest of the individual patient, that in difficult cases he may have the advantages of the highest skill available, and secondly in the interest of the medical men attached to the Primary and Secondary Centres, that they may have the opportunity to fol- low the later stages of an illness in which they have been concerned at the beginning, to make themselves acquainted with the treatment adopted, and to appreciate the needs of a patient after his return home.

---

1. Numbers refer to paragraph numbers in the Dawson Report.

The Dawson Report went into much more detail, describing the
services of the three levels of health centers as well as supple-
mentary services. Concern was also expressed for establishing
the necessary relationships among the several levels.

> 93. It is vital to the success of any scheme of Health
> Service that there should be unity of idea and purpose, and
> complete and reciprocal communication between the associated
> Teaching Hospitals, Secondary Health Centres, Primary Health
> Centres, and the Domiciliary Services, whether the Centres
> are situated in town or country.

The report noted that existing methods of health administration would not achieve the desired results and called for "a new
type of Health Authority to bring about unity of local control for
all health services, curative and preventive." The counselors,
however, were not ready to specify the nature of the new Health
Authority but said,

> 95. Whatever may be the nature of the future Health
> Authority, it will be necessary to devise machinery for
> securing the complete intercommunication and co-ordination
> above referred to, and what we desire to emphasize here is
> that such intercommunication is vital to an efficient health
> organization.

Committee on the Costs of Medical Care. In the United States, the
28 reports of the Committee on the Costs of Medical Care (the
final report was issued in 1932) are regarded as landmark docu-
ments. They covered a wide range of topics, but there was a
strong emphasis on the organization of the health care system.
Provocative at the time was the committee's advocacy of organized
hospital-based group practices. The committee also presented a
plan that contained the major elements of a regionalized program
of personal health services. "Its scheme began with the philosophy that the keystone of the concept of a satisfactory medical
service for the nation is development of one or more nonprofit
"community health centers" in nearly every city of approximately
15,000 population or more. Community medical centers would super-
vise various branches and medical stations. It is this characteristic of coordinated, decentralized services with a two-way
flow of patient care which associates the proposal with regional
medical care" (Pearson, 1976).

Hospital Survey and Construction Act (Hill-Burton). Regionaliza-
tion received renewed interest and support during and immediately
following World War II. In 1943 the Subcommittee on Wartime
Health and Education of the Senate Committee on Education and
Labor was established. In hearings of the subcommittee in 1944,
Thomas Parran, Surgeon General of the U.S. Public Health Service
(USPHS), expressed the thinking of the Public Health Service about
a number of issues including the equitable distribution of hospi-

tals. Notable in this work were the efforts of Joseph W. Mountin
of the USPHS, who along with others developed a conceptual model
based on empirical research of hospital service areas. Figure 4.1
appeared in the U.S. Public Health Service publication, "Health
Service Areas: Requirements for General Hospitals and Health
Centers," by Mountin et al. The publication set forth a plan
whereby health centers and small hospitals would be coordinated
with larger hospitals. Health centers were to provide general
medical care for ambulatory patients and preventive health services. There would be free interchange among the units, and persons entering a health center would have at their disposal all the
resources of the medical service area. The effort of the Subcommittee on Wartime Health and Education and the work of the USPHS,
especially that of Joseph Mountin, influenced the passage of
federal legislation for the support of hospital construction--the
Hospital Survey and Construction Act of 1946 (Hill-Burton Act).
This legislation required that each state survey its hospital
needs and prepare a state plan for future development, following
quite closely the idea of service areas and the location of hospitals based on the Public Health Service model.
     The Hill-Burton legislation has greatly influenced hospital

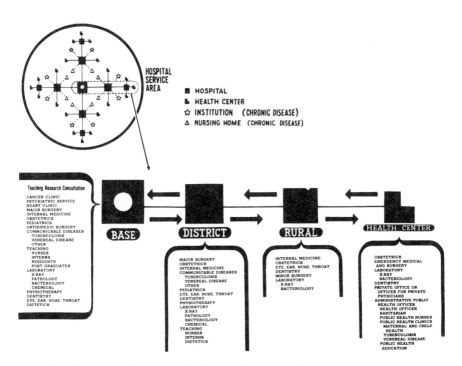

Fig. 4.1. A diagram showing relationships among base,
           district, and rural hospitals and health centers
           in a coordinated service plan.

construction in rural areas. In reviewing its effects, Milton
Roemer (1976a) points out that the legislation provided for construction in areas of greatest need based on surveys in each
state. Inevitably this meant that more aid went to rural areas,
greatly improving rural hospital facilities. Between 1946 and
1966 the disparity in number of hospital beds between predominantly rural and urban states was almost eliminated. However,
although some rationality was achieved in the location of hospitals, organizational coordination among them was not achieved.

Commission on Hospital Care. Development and passage of the Hill-
Burton legislation cannot be attributed entirely to efforts of the
USPHS or to the committees of Congress. Influence also came from
the American Hospital Association and various foundations in their
support of the Commission on Hospital Care. The planning committee for the commission, formed in 1942, was chaired by Graham L.
Davis, director of the Kellogg Foundation. The commission recommended regional coordination of hospital services, which paral-
leled the recommendations of Joseph Mountin and others of the
USPHS. It advocated regional hospital plans, citing as exemplary
the Rochester Regional Hospital Council and the Bingham Associates
Fund program, the latter establishing linkages between hospitals
in small towns in Maine and a medical center in Boston. Through
efforts of the commission and state hospital associations a series
of inventories of facilities was undertaken. Pearson (1976) says,
"One of the Commission's major concerns was national planning for
health services through regional hospital care, and it suggested
that each state be divided into hospital regions, with each region
centered around one or more major regional hospitals. Community
hospitals would be located within well-defined trade areas, which
would be established according to marketing research methods."
Roemer notes that the commission's report in 1946, together with
the work of the USPHS, laid the technical basis for the Hill-
Burton legislation (Roemer, 1976a).
    Dan Feshbach (1979), in a review of the legislative history
of Hill-Burton, contends that the role of the Kellogg Foundation
in the Commission on Hospital Care, through the participation of
its director, Graham L. Davis, biased the legislation toward rural
areas. Feshbach also contends that Hill-Burton was a response of
the health care establishment, which the Commission on Hospital
Care represented, to the threat of national health insurance.

Other reports. Reports of commissions, studies by foundations,
and activities by states in planning and organizing health activities continued to be made and in them advocacy of regionalization
had become standard. Clearly, the Ewing Report (Ewing, 1948) and
the Magnuson Commission Report (Magnuson, 1952) were in this vein.
Pearson (1976) made the following comments on the Magnuson Commission Report.

    The Magnuson Commission takes on added interest from the

fact that its report was published five years after the report of the Commission on Hospital Care, six years after the
passage of the Hospital Survey and Construction Act, and
twenty years after the landmark recommendations of the Committee on the Costs of Medical Care. The recommendations of
all these groups are parallel regarding medical care regionalization. However, because progress in implementing regional concepts was slow, the Magnuson Commission obviously
felt it necessary to repeat previously identified regional
concepts.

Recent and Present Programs in Regionalization

Regional Medical Programs. In spite of support for regionalization in reports of government, foundations, and professional societies, serious efforts to implement regionalized programs by the
federal government, aside from the Hill-Burton program, were not
made until the 1960s. Regional Medical Programs (RMP) was the
name given to an effort which may be viewed as the first federal
effort explicitly designed to impose specific principles of organization upon the general health care system (Ostow and Brudney,
1977). RMP did not succeed. It was altered, perhaps fatally,
from its original conception and then oversold and underfinanced.
Its impact on the health of the nation could not be demonstrated,
but it is worth considering for its intent and for its portent.
The impetus for Regional Medical Programs came from the report of the President's Commission on Heart Disease, Cancer, and
Stroke--1964, Michael DeBakey, chairman.

> The first major proposal was for the five-year development of
> a network of regional medical centers for each of the major
> categories (heart disease, cancer, and stroke) for investiga-
> tion, teaching and patient care. At the community level, a
> second diagnostic and treatment network for patient care was
> formulated. In terms of revising interinstitutional rela-
> tionships (the essence of functional regionalization), the
> most significant contribution of the report was the proposed
> formation of 30 regional medical complexes to coordinate
> university medical schools, hospitals, and other health in-
> stitutions [Ostow and Brudney, 1977].

RMP in this version clearly would have restructured the
health delivery system by placing medical centers at schools of
medicine at the apex of a coordinated health care system. Such a
development was, as might be expected, viewed with alarm by
organized medicine. Through effective lobbying, the opposition
was able to constrain the universities' encroachment into the
health delivery system. The RMP legislation was, Ostow and
Brudney (1977) say, "shorn of most of the features that might have
achieved any significant degree of regionalization. The categori-
cal emphasis (heart disease, cancer, and stroke) was reinforced,

the provision for the development of therapeutic stations was
eliminated, voluntary interinstitutional cooperation replaced
facilities coordination, and the interests of the private practitioner were protected. Continuing education and training were
emphasized relative to reorganization of service delivery." In
the statement of the legislation, the program was specifically
prohibited from "interfering with the patterns, or the methods of
financing, of patient care or professional practice or with the
administration of hospitals. . . . No patient shall be furnished
hospital, medical, or other care . . . unless he has been referred
. . . by a practicing physician" (PL 89-239).

     Thus RMP emphasized continuing education and information dis-
semination. Its research and demonstration projects tended to be
noncumulative and had little impact. By 1973, RMP was slated for
extinction but lingered until it was superseded by the National
Health Planning and Resources Development Act of 1974 (PL 93-641).

Comprehensive Health Planning. Comprehensive Health Planning
(CHP) is often mentioned as a companion program to RMP. Although
these two programs existed simultaneously and both were efforts by
the federal government to rationalize the health delivery system,
they were not coordinated with each other and often contended for
resources and attention. The competition reflected the constit-
uency of the respective programs, with RMP being university-
centered while CHP was in the political-action arena.

     The legislation creating CHP stated, "Comprehensive health
planning is viewed as a process that will enable rational decision-making about the use of public and private resources to meet
health needs. Its concern encompasses physical, mental, and en-
vironmental health; the facilities, services, and manpower required to meet all health needs; and the development and coordination of public, voluntary, and private resources to meet these
needs" (PL 89-749).

     The legislation authorized the establishment and funding of
state and substate planning agencies. The statewide agencies
known as CHP "a" agencies dealt with long-range planning and the
allocation of federal monies. The objective was to utilize planning to achieve rational regionalization (Decker, 1977). The substate area agencies known as CHP "b" agencies were involved in
local planning and day-to-day decisions. Of interest is that a
majority of consumers was required on the governing boards of each
of the agencies.

     As with RMP, CHP did not fulfill its promise. Characteris-
tically, the "b" agencies became bogged down in data collection
and the time-consuming task of review and comment on grant applications of local providers to the federal government. In reviewing the accomplishments of CHP, Decker points out that there was
an inadequate supply of trained planning staff members to contend
with the "giants of local medicine." Also, the development dol-
lars it controlled were small when compared with the amounts spent
by the federal government and the private sector in direct health

services--Decker likens it to ants against elephants. He concludes that CHP never had the leverage to influence significantly
the health delivery system and furthermore, it became politicized
and was relatively easy for a strong minority of health care providers to dominate. "Providers essentially sought decentralization and individual institutional objectives and thus made rationalization of the health delivery system by CHP impossible"
(Decker, 1977).

National Health Planning and Resources Development Act. The Na-
tional Health Planning and Resources Development Act of 1974 (PL
93-641) superseded or took over some of the activities of the
Hill-Burton program and RMP, but its most direct ancestor was ·CHP.
In this program at the state level are State Health Planning and
Development Agencies (SHPDAs) and Statewide Health Coordinating
Councils (SHCCs); at the substate level are Health System Agencies
(HSAs). SHPDAs and HSAs conform in many ways to the CHP "a" and
"b" agencies respectively and often are staffed by the same personnel. This legislation, however, gives the planning agencies
more power and represents a second generation of health planning.
     Some 200 HSAs are the building blocks of the health planning
system. Governors of states designate Health Service Areas, which
with some exceptions are between 500,000 and 3 million in population. The governing bodies of HSAs are, by statute, composed of
10 to 30 members (except they may be larger in the cases where
there is an executive committee--a situation that tends to be the
rule), of whom a majority but not more than 60 percent are consumers and the remainder are providers of health services. The
provision is also made that the consumers are to be broadly representative of the social, economic, linguistic, and racial populations; geographic areas; and major purchasers of health care.
HSAs have the responsibility to prepare long-range health service
plans and annual implementation plans for the area. This involves
inventories and analyses of number, type, and location of the
area's health resources. The plans of the agency must be consistent with the standards set forth in the National Guidelines for
Health Planning of the Department of Health and Human Services
(HHS). HSAs have some power to influence the development of
health facilities and programs in their areas. The legislation
mandates states to enact certificate-of-need legislation that en-
ables HSAs to review, with power of approval, the development and
expansion of facilities in their areas (final approval is by
SHPDA). HSAs also have review and approval power over Public
Health Service funds and federal grants used to support the development of health resources in the area.
     At the state level SHPDAs are units of state government
designated by the governors with HHS agreement. The companion
public board is the State Health Coordinating Council (SHCC). The
state agency must have an administrative program and prepare an
annual preliminary State Health Plan which takes into account the
plans of HSAs and is submitted to the SHCC. SHPDAs serve as

1122 agencies,[2] administer the state certificate-of-need program, and review (with SHCCs) the State Medical Facilities plan (formerly Hill-Burton).

The composition of SHCCs, by statute, consists of not less than 16 members appointed by the governor from nominees submitted by HSAs, not less than half of whom are consumers. The governor may appoint additional members (non-HSA nominees), but they are not to exceed 40 percent of the total membership, with a majority being consumers. The main function of the SHCCs is to review and coordinate long-range and annual implementation plans of HSAs and to prepare the annual State Health Plan in conjunction with SHPDAs.

The greater effectiveness of current planning comes not only from its "teeth" in the form of review and approval powers but also from the urgent need for cost containment. It is thought that by eliminating duplication of services and limiting health facility construction, savings can be made in the cost of health care. For this reason, health planning caught the attention of corporate enterprise whose costs for employee health fringe benefits are substantial. Another advantage that the present program has over its predecessor is a cadre of trained and more experienced health planners who are better able to hold their own in encounters with the private medical establishment. The latter point appears to be crucial. Basil Mott (1977) says,

> The rhetoric of planning is one of rational decision making, but health planning is more political than technological, since there is so little basis for rational action. The central issues are questions of values and interests, such as whether everyone should have equal access to health care or whether some inequality should be tolerated in order to devote more national resources to other social needs. These questions cannot be settled objectively through technology. In a situation where no party can dictate, problems can be settled only through processes of conflict and bargaining.

Health planning is needed in the federal government's involvement in the delivery of personal health services. The guidelines for health planning emphasize cost containment through such mechanisms as establishing standards for the ratio of hospital beds to population, hospital occupancy rates, and minimum numbers of certain procedures. For example, the guidelines set forth the standards that there should be less than four nonfederal, short-stay hospital beds for each 1,000 persons in a health service area

---

2. Agencies authorized by the 1972 amendment (section 1122) to the Social Security Act, which gives state planning agencies power to approve or reject proposals to expand specified services or facilities. The capital expenditures include those that exceed $100,000, those that change the bed capacity of the facility, and those that change the services of the facility.

except under extraordinary circumstances; that there should be an average annual occupancy rate of medically necessary hospital care of at least 80 percent for all nonfederal, short-stay hospital beds considered together in a service area except under extraordinary circumstances; and that within three years after initiation there should be a minimum of 200 open heart procedures performed annually in any institution in which open heart surgery is performed for adults.

The legislation itself does not expressly mandate regionalization of health services. Karl Yordy (1976), in a careful review of PL 93-641, found that the term "regionalization" did not appear in the legislation, although certain of the National Health Priorities (section 1502 of the legislation) are supportive of the concept. It is in the National Guidelines for Health Planning that the concept is made explicit and in a sense operational for health planning. In view of this, it is instructive to examine in more detail the guidelines for one type of service that illustrates the emphasis on regionalization of services and exercise of control. The entry in the Guideline for Neonatal Special Care Units is as follows:[3]

121.204--Neonatal Special Care Units
(a) Standard
  (1) Neonatal services should be planned on a regional basis with linkages with obstetrical services.
  (2) The total number of neonatal intensive and intermediate care beds should not exceed 4 per 1,000 live births per year in a defined neonatal service area. An adjustment upward may be justified when the rate of high-risk pregnancies is unusually high, based on analyses by the HSA.
  (3) A single neonatal special care unit (Level II or III) should contain a minimum of 15 beds. An adjustment downward may be justified for a Level II unit when travel time to an alternative unit is a serious hardship due to geographic remoteness, based on analyses by HSA.
(b) Discussion--For this standard, the Department has adopted the widely endorsed concept of regionalization, involving various levels of care. Under this concept,

----

   3. In addition to Standards for Neonatal Special Care Units, "Standards Respecting the Appropriate Supply, Distribution, and Organization of Health Resources" are developed for: General Hospitals--Bed Supply; General Hospitals--Occupancy Rate; Obstetrical Services; Pediatric Inpatient Services--Number of Beds; Pediatric Inpatient Services--Occupancy Rates; Open Heart Surgery; Cardiac Catheterization; Radiation Therapy; Computed Tomographic Scanners; End-State Renal Disease (National Health Guidelines, USDHEW Publ. HRA 78-643).

Level III units are staffed and equipped for the intensive care of new-borns as well as intermediate and recovery care. Level II units provide intermediate and recovery care as well as some specialized services. Level I units provide recovery care. Neonatal special care is highly specialized service required by only a very small percentage of infants. The Department believes that four neonatal special care beds for intensive and intermediate care per 1,000 live births will usually be adequate to meet the needs, taking into account the incidence of high risk pregnancies, the percentage of live births requiring intensive care, and the average length of stay. ("Bed" includes incubators or other heated units for specialized care, and bassinets.) In addition, the Department has established a minimum of 15 beds per unit for Levels II and III as the minimum number necessary to support economical operation for these services. Both standards are supported and recommended by the American Academy of Pediatrics.

The American Academy of Pediatrics has noted that "the best care will be given to high risk and seriously ill neonates if intensive care units are developed in a few adequately qualified institutions within a community rather than within many hospitals. Properly conducted, early transfer of these infants to a qualified unit provides better care than do attempts to maintain them in inadequate units." This regionalization approach is reflected in the minimum size standard which is designed to foster the location of specialized units of medical centers which have available special staff, equipment, and consultative services and facilities.

Since prenatal centers which include neonatal units will serve the patient load resulting from a representative population of more than one million, a defined neonatal service area should be identified by the relevant HSAs in conjunction with the State Agency. Special attention should also be given to ensure adequate communication and transportation systems, including joint transfers of mother and child and maintenance of family contact. Hospitals with such units should have agreements with other facilities to serve referred patients. The regional plan should include a structured ongoing system of review, including assessment of changes in health status indicators [USDHEW, 1978a].

PL 93-641 has some special implications for rural areas. Certain exceptions are made in standards in level of utilization, minimum size of facilities, and quantity of services per capita (i.e., hospital beds per 1,000 population). The exceptions are commonly related to density of population and thus to the rural population. Furthermore, consumer membership on HSA governing boards is to be allocated according to characteristics of the pop-

ulation, with metropolitan-nonmetropolitan specified as one of the
characteristics to be considered. But more importantly, to the
extent that the planning mandate is carried out, rural areas are
brought into a regionalized system of health services.

Rural Health Initiative. The Rural Health Initiative (RHI) is a
program directed specifically to rural areas. Its statements of
goals embrace regionalization. RHI was established in 1975 in the
Bureau of Community Health Services of the U.S. Public Health
Service as an administrative effort to integrate a number of
existing federal health programs and to assist in the development
of health care systems for rural areas. Existing programs include: National Health Services Corps Program, Migrant Health
Program, Community Health Centers Program, and Appalachian Health
Program. All of the program resources may be used, together with
other federal programs, to develop rural health care systems.
Such systems should also be coordinated with local resources such
as home health services, school health services, and local transportation services (USDHEW, 1978b).
    The introductory remarks in the Rural Health Initiative
Program Guidance Material say,

> Experience over the past few years indicates that the most
> feasible solution to problems in rural health care lies in
> the establishment of rural systems of health care delivery.
> A health care system should attempt to meet the health needs
> of all people. A complete health care system is comprised of
> primary, secondary and tertiary care. . . . Primary (basic)
> health care can be provided on an ambulatory or walk-in basis
> within reasonable distance of those being served. Some
> patients will need specialty care and hospitalization (sec-
> ondary care), and some may need the more specialized diagnos-
> tic services or treatment (such as heart surgery) available
> only in large medical centers (tertiary care). Therefore,
> for a primary health care system to be complete, it must pro-
> vide access to secondary and tertiary care. Such access is
> arranged by the primary care provider, who has established
> contacts with appropriate secondary and tertiary care pro-
> viders. Those contacts that have been pre-established by
> phone, letter, or personal conferences will permit referrals
> of patients appropriately and promptly [USDHEW, 1978b].

    In conjunction with the above statement, a diagram of a model
health care is presented (Fig. 4.2). Although it is drawn somewhat differently, in content it is similar to the model that
Joseph Mountin developed for the Hill-Burton program and very
close to the concept of regionalization presented in the Dawson
Report.

Emergency Medical Services. Emergency Medical Services (EMS)
should lend themselves to regionalization. The need to provide

appropriate levels of service and reliable and prompt transportation in emergency situations is compelling. It is easy to visualize a hierarchy of EMS units (hospital emergency departments of
different levels of sophistication) and a technology of communication and transportation that links them together to provide fast,
reliable, and appropriate services in medical emergencies. The
federal government has intervened more directly in the delivery of
emergency medical services with both criteria and resources than
in any other area of health delivery.

The first major effort was through the Highway Safety Act of
1966, which was administered by the Department of Transportation.
The legislation required that states develop EMS programs as a

A Stratified Health System

**TERTIARY MEDICAL CARE AND HEALTH SERVICES:
FOR A STATE OR MULTIPLE COUNTY REGION**

(Provided in a Medical Center of a University Teaching Center)

Quality specialty care in a personalized fashion:

1. Specialized medical, diagnostic, and therapeutic services for unusual and complicated cases.
2. Specialized surgical care for unusual and complicated
cases (neurosurgery, organ transplants, etc.)
3. Specialized dental care for unusual and complicated
oral disease and surgery.
4. Emergency medical care.
5. Part of a comprehensive health care system.

**SECONDARY MEDICAL CARE AND HEALTH SERVICES:
FOR A REGION**

(Provided in a Regional Hospital or Health Center)

Quality secondary and referral care in an available and personalized fashion:

1. Medical and surgical diagnostic services for complicated
problems.
2. Surgical care and medical care for complicated problems.
3. Services for major surgical and medical emergency problems.
4. Specialty dental care—orthodontics, endodontics, periodontics.
5. Emergency medical care.
6. Part of a comprehensive health care system.

**PRIMARY MEDICAL CARE AND HEALTH SERVICES:
FOR AN AREA**

(Provided in an Area Health Ambulatory Center)

Quality primary care and health services in an available, personalized, and
continuous fashion:

1. Preventive services, case-finding services, and diagnosis and treatment for
usual and uncomplicated illness and disease.
2. Minor surgery and medical care for uncomplicated problems.
3. Home care programs—nursing services.
4. Preventive, diagnostic, and restorative dental services.
5. Part of a comprehensive health care system.
6. (In large Area Health Centers, services for surgical and medical problems
not requiring specialized personnel and equipment.)

(Provided in a Community Health Center, usually a satellite to an Area
Primary Health Center)

Quality primary medical care and health services in an available, personalized, and continuous fashion:

1. Preventive services, case finding services, and diagnosis and treatment for
usual and uncomplicated illness and disease.
2. Supervision of home care health services.
3. Part of the comprehensive health care system.

Fig. 4.2. A stratified health system.

condition for obtaining federal highway construction funds. Quite
specific standards were stated involving the training of personnel, type of emergency vehicles, communication system, dispatching
system, and development of comprehensive emergency plans (Gibson,
1977a). Not all states complied with the requirements of the
legislation; even so, the sanction of withholding highway construction funds was never used.

The Department of Health, Education and Welfare entered the
local EMS programs through the mechanisms of Regional Medical
Programs and Comprehensive Health Planning, but the projects
funded under these mechanisms were diffused and fragmented. Following this, a major demonstration was undertaken in which substantial resources were committed to statewide programs in Arkansas and Illinois and to area programs in rural Ohio, in and around
San Diego, California, and in Jacksonville, Florida. Before the
results of the demonstrations were in, however, Congress passed
the Emergency Medical Services Systems Act of 1973 (PL 93-154).
The program guidelines for implementation of the legislation take
a thoroughly regionalized stance, which is reflected in 15 mandatory requirements for local funding.

A major means of achieving regionalization is through the
communication system. The guidelines state:

> Provisions for linking the personnel, facilities, and equip-
> ment of the systems by a central communications facility
> which 1) utilizes emergency telephonic screening, 2) utilizes
> or will utilize the universal telephone number 911, and 3)
> will have direct communication connections and interconnec-
> tions with the personnel, facilities, and equipment of the
> system with other appropriate emergency medical service sys-
> tems [Gibson, 1977b].

The guideline standards also call for providing access to
emergency facilities that have appropriate standards with regard
to capacity, location, personnel, and equipment and that are coordinated with other health facilities of the system. There should
also be access to specialized critical medical care units. The
major problem addressed here is the appropriate use of emergency
medical facilities within an area. Gibson (1977b) says,

> The strategy for the future would reduce the current mismatch
> between resources available and resources clinically needed
> by rerouting emergency department patients to the most
> appropriate treatment facility. Ambulance systems have been
> criticized for taking patients not to the most appropriate
> hospital but to the nearest facility where, for example, they
> may wait up to 30 minutes for the physician on call. Highly
> specialized trauma centers at large teaching hospitals are
> often under utilized because trauma patients are taken to
> small, ill-equipped community hospitals. Well-staffed and
> well-equipped large emergency departments often treat fewer

critically ill patients than smaller less adequate emergency
rooms.
The solution to the problem offered by the profession is categorization of hospital emergency services, designating the relative preparedness and capabilities of hospitals and their staffs
to provide emergency medical care. In 1971, the AMA Commission on
Emergency Medical Services sponsored a multidisciplinary conference on Categorization of Hospital Emergency Services.[4] EMS were
categorized into four levels of specialization from lowest level
IV (Basic Emergency Service Capabilities) to highest level I (Comprehensive Emergency Service Capabilities). The commission specified in detail the character of staff, facilities, and equipment
both for the emergency department and for the hospital (Hampton,
1976).

Geoffrey Gibson (1977b) says, "EMS health planning activities
throughout the Nation are predominantly based on the categorization, both as a strategy for change and as a method for assessing
the adequacy of the present EMS system." In general, Gibson concludes that categorization has not achieved regionalization of
emergency services.

> While it is relatively easy to attach descriptive labels to
> the variable capacities of hospitals to render emergency
> care, it is almost insuperably difficult to implement such
> categorization by altering patient and ambulance utilization
> patterns. For categorization to have any impact on where
> patients are treated it must, of course, alter present care
> patterns; certain high-risk conditions should be rerouted
> from smaller community hospitals to larger teaching specialty
> centers.
>   The reaction of community hospitals has in most juris-
> dictions been hostile, deeply felt, and successful. The ad-
> ministrators have pointed out that since approximately one-
> third of all inpatient days are generated through the emer-
> gency department, which also makes a twenty-four hour provi-
> sion of ancillary services fiscally viable, a rerouting of
> high-risk patients (most likely to be admitted) from commu-
> nity to teaching hospitals would have a devastating financial
> impact on the former. Similarly, the medical staffs at com-
> munity hospitals have also resisted categorization, since it
> may well prevent their caring for their private patients at
> their usual hospital. Faced with this reaction, local EMS
> systems have experienced severe difficulty in implementing
> federal mandates for facility and critical care unit region-
> alized planning [Gibson, 1977a].

---

4. Other participants were the American College of Surgeons,
the American Academy of Orthopaedic Surgeons, the American Society
of Anesthesiologists, the American Academy of Pediatrics, and the
National Academy of Sciences-National Research Council.

Regionalization Related to Performance

The ultimate argument for regionalization is improvement of performance. The assumption is made, for example, that a surgical team needs to perform a minimum number of procedures in a year in order to maintain high quality skills. Harold Luft et al. (1979) provide some systematic evidence in this regard. In their research they examined mortality rates for 12 surgical procedures of varying complexity in 1,498 hospitals to determine whether there is a relationship between a hospital's surgical volume and its surgical mortality. They found that for certain more complicated procedures there was a lower mortality rate with greater volume of surgery. For open-heart surgery, transurethral resection of the prostate, and coronary bypasses, hospitals in which 200 or more of these operations were done annually had death rates (adjusted for case mix) 25 to 41 percent lower than hospitals with lower volumes. For other procedures the mortality curve flattened out at lower volumes. For example, hospitals doing 50 to 100 total hip replacements attained a mortality rate almost as low as that for hospitals doing 200 or more. Other procedures such as cholecystectomies and vagotomies showed no relationship between volume and mortality. In general the authors interpreted their data as supporting regionalization as a means of improving performance. They say that rather than concentrating all surgery in a few large-scale medical centers, regionalization may be achieved by having moderate-sized and smaller hospitals doing safer and volume-insensitive procedures. "Thus, although regionalization may require a substantial improvement in the referral patterns for certain, more complex procedures, it is possible that large segments of surgical practice may not require change" (Luft et al., 1979).

In a subsequent issue of the *New England Journal of Medicine*, however, Murray Feldstein (1980) takes issue with Luft et al. He maintains that to ascertain the value of regionalization one would have to know the adverse effects of regionalization in a larger context and subtract them from the anticipated gains. For example, centralization of the most complex procedures might result in relocation of specialists to the detriment of some communities. The dangers of traveling to centers should be taken into account. Furthermore, centralization would magnify the possible incompetence of a particular surgeon or surgical team.

Much agreement exists on the form a regionalized health services system would take. There is substantial support for establishing regionalized systems as a means of efficiently delivering high quality health services. However, application has been halting. A major question is how the system should be controlled. At one extreme are those who advocate controls of the marketplace and professional relations. At the other extreme are those who advocate centralized control with corporate managers and administrative apparatus. The following chapter deals with the implications of different modes of control for the organization of health services.

Control Processes in Regionalized Interorganizational Fields

Regionalization represents a special type of interorganizational field. In it different levels of services are provided, services are distributed spatially, and they are integrated through some type of "control" process. The control process may range from interorganizational exchanges of the marketplace to the bureaucratic structure of the planning agency. These processes are discussed by a number of analysts who emphasize different aspects of the situation but converge at certain points.

Robert Alford uses the concept of structural interests in the health care field. Structural interests are defined in terms of their relationship (fit) to existing institutions of the society and are classified as dominant, challenging, and repressed. The dominant structural interests in medical care are *professional monopolists* headed by physicians and biomedical researchers.

> Medicine is a classic case of social organization of production but the private appropriation of powers and benefits by a structural interest--professional monopoly--which through professional associations has maintained control of the supply of physicians, the distribution of cost of services, and the rules governing hospitals [Alford, 1975].

The challenge to professional monopoly comes from *corporate rationalization*. Alford points out that the organization of health care has become increasingly social and involves a complex division of labor between skilled persons specializing in primary care, surgery, preventive medicine, and other areas. Hospitals, bureaucratically structured, are the principal agents available to organize this complex of technology and skilled personnel.

While the professional monopolists and corporate rationalists participate in a common institutional milieu, the "outsider" structure (repressed structural interests) is represented in Alford's typology as community population structural interests. As illustrative but not exhaustive of interest groups in the community structure, Alford lists white rural and urban poor, ghetto

blacks, lower middle class just above the Medicaid income maximum,
neighborhoods just poor enough that no doctor wants to establish
his practice there, middle-class families rendered newly medically
indigent by sharply escalating costs, and those in occupations
affected by job-related diseases. The key difference between dominant and repressed structural interests is that "enormous political and organizational energies must be summoned by repressed
structural interests to offset the intrinsic disadvantages of
their situation. None need be generated by dominant structural
interests" (Alford, 1975). The reality of this distinction can be
seen by anyone observing the small gains made by community groups
in changing the health care system only to see them melt away,
encapsulated, or absorbed into the dominant health care system.

The actual contention in the health care system is between
the dominant professional monopolists and the challenging corporate rationalists.

> The pluralist view [representing that of the professional
> monopolist] emphasizes the need for the autonomy of all of
> the elements of the health care system--the doctors, the hos-
> pitals, the researchers, the medical schools--and opposes a
> general program of rationalization and subsidy by the govern-
> ment because it will interfere with the operations of a com-
> petitive market in health care. Such a market, it is
> claimed, will drive out the inefficient producers and make
> the remaining producers more responsive to consumer demand.
> The bureaucratic view [representing that of the corporate ra-
> tionalists], on the other hand, emphasizes the need for inte-
> gration of all of the same elements, in order to overcome
> duplication (which the pluralists hail as diversity), lack of
> coordination (which the pluralists welcome as competition),
> and lack of planning (which the pluralists condemn as both
> unnecessary and impossible) [Alford, 1975].

Alford seeks evidence of the relationship between the dominant structural interests (professional monopolists) and their
challengers (corporate rationalists) in a detailed analysis of
reports of various health commissions of New York City. He concludes that the study-planning activity can be subverted. Instead of being a step in the process of rationalization of health
care delivery it becomes a mechanism to delay actions and maintain the status quo.

> Planning becomes holding meetings, consulting, and communi-
> cating, not hard analysis of empirical data on the conse-
> quences of alternative policy decisions.
>
> The very mechanisms which are intended to insure plan-
> ning guarantee that no planning takes place. The mechanisms
> of coordination become instruments of the status quo. And
> this is by no means accidental. The major parties to these
> investigations, councils, and commissions do not intend to

"change the system." They wish to reinforce it, or at the most to allow only a little change--a few more hospitals will be constructed, affiliation of a clinic or hospital with a medical school will be achieved, a nursing program will begin [Alford, 1975].

David Pearson, in his historical review of regionalization in the United States, was able to discern two distinct models of regionalization which give support to Alford's conceptualization. One model concentrates on *direct patient care*, the other on *planning and coordination* of services. The former is more tightly organized and authoritatively controlled, the latter depends on voluntary controls. The direct patient care model overlaps Alford's corporate rationalization, while the planning and coordination model overlaps his professional monopolist model. Pearson (1976) perceives (as does Alford) that the direct care model is a challenge to professional health practitioners:

> Basically, the patient care model proposes an authoritative and structured approach to regionalization, while the planning and coordination model emphasizes voluntary participation and cooperation. The patient care model requires a dramatic change in the organization of medical care. Those opposing such a change appear to have proposed the planning and coordination model as an alternative to the proposals that focused on integrating personal health services. What is seen, therefore, is an example of social policy competition between idealists, who perceived the need of a dramatic change in structuring the delivery of comprehensive medical care, and pragmatists, who could not accept the breadth and depth of the proposals.

CONTROL CONFIGURATIONS

Edward Lehman has developed a typology of organizational relationships based on *control configurations* that characterize different organizational fields. The work is prior to that of Alford's and compatible with it at a number of points. The typology is a value-added construct in that "(1) the configurations listed first are more 'simple' and reflect less conscious control of an interorganizational field, while subsequent ones are progressively more 'complex' and contain more deliberate patterns of control; and (2) each succeeding pattern contains all the elements of the preceding ones plus at least one 'added' factor" (Lehman, 1975).

Three broad patterns of control are identified as (1) a field of laterally linked organizations--termed a feudal field, (2) mediated interorganizational relationships, and (3) guided interorganizational relationships. The last of these patterns is divided between an interorganizational field dominated by a single member--termed an empire--and an administered interorganizational field--termed a corporate guided field. The factors on which the types vary are:

(1) the degree to which interorganizational contacts entail procedures to inform or to consult one another versus the degree to which such contacts entail arrangements for actual co-decision-making about the future state of the field; (2) the degree to which the resources necessary for the wielding of systemic power (that is, for deciding upon joint goals, for pursuing them, and for implementing them) remain in the hands of the member organizations; and (3) the extent to which the responsibility for wielding systemic power is attributed to the individual member organizations versus the extent to which it is centered in an agency acting in the name of the entire field [Lehman, 1975].

The typology also specifically considers differential authority and power in interorganizational fields. Thus it provides for progression from the pluralism of market economy decision making to the centrality of political economy decision making. Characteristics of the types are presented below.

Laterally Linked Fields--Interorganizational Feudalism
Lehman (1975) suggests an analogy between this type of interorganizational field and European feudal societies.

In these systems, the foci of identification and integration of member units (for example, fiefs, baronies, duchies, and so on) were largely internal rather than directed toward some center of systemic power. Furthermore, such systems lacked a strong controlling overlayer (for example, a Napoleonic state) that could exercise effective systemic power in either the market or political sector. Even where there was some collectivity-orientation, both responsibility for wielding systemic power and the control of requisite resources tended to be localized largely in the member units themselves [Lehman, 1975].

In laterally linked fields in health care delivery, (1) activity is oriented to information exchange and consultation rather than joint decision making, (2) control of the fields is retained by member units and resources, and (3) power is dispersed among the administrative centers of the member organizations. Lehman identifies Levine's and White's work on interorganizational exchange among health agencies in a community of 200,000 population in New England as a classic study of a feudalistic configuration. The data indicated that this research site could be characterized as "a field of largely autonomous organizations whose interactions were determined by mutual self-interest and were direct--that is,

were neither mediated or guided" (Lehman, 1975). All units in a
laterally linked system are not equal, however, and patterns of
dominance and subordination do emerge in a field.

The large number of different types of health service units
is evident to the most casual observer, including hospitals, nursing homes, home nursing units, clinics, physicians' office practices, and public health departments. The list could be greatly
extended and much more detailed. For example, physicians' office
practices could be identified according to specialization and to
solo and/or type of group.

Sol Levine and Paul White (1961) have advanced our understanding of interrelationships among health service units. While
each health organization has its own goals and must pursue them
successfully in order to survive, it also requires resources from
its environment. Resources that service-type groups usually need
are clients, skilled personnel, material items including money,
information, and knowledge. Principal elements in the environment
are other health service units. An important source of resources
comes from *exchange* with other health service units.

A characteristic of exchange relationships is that they are
mutually beneficial to the parties involved; thus physicians in
private office practice engage in exchange relationships with hospitals to the benefit of both. The principal source of clients
for hospitals is admission by private physicians. And private
physicians provide expertise in caring for hospitalized patients.
The hospital assembles the technology and personnel essential to
the physician's practice. It is commonly pointed out that hospital facilities are essential in attracting physicians to rural
areas. It is equally true that physicians are necessary to fill
hospital beds and hospital administrators are among the most dili-
gent recruiters of physicians in rural areas. Their purpose is to
maintain hospital bed censuses in rural hospitals, which is a
chronic problem.

A mutually beneficial relationship may occur between short-
term hospitals and long-term care facilities such as nursing homes.
Long-term facilities relieve the hospital of care for low revenue
producing patients who cannot benefit from intensive treatment,
and short-term hospitals provide clients to long-term facilities.
Exchange between the short-term hospital and the Visiting Nurses
Association program is mutually beneficial in a similar way.

Differentiation on the basis of levels of service (i.e.,
specialization among physicians or the more general primary, secondary, and tertiary categorization) clearly suggests *exchange*
among units. Referral of patients is a major mechanism of exchange, with certain specialists highly dependent on referrals
from other physicians, and tertiary health care units dependent on
primary and secondary level units for patients. The benefits
returning to primary level units are the expertise of consulting
personnel and the technology unavailable at lower-level units.
Furthermore, it is common for tertiary units such as comprehensive

cancer centers to provide educational experiences for staffs in
secondary and primary centers (in exchange for channeling patients
to them).

In view of these kinds of relationships, Levine et al. (1963)
chose the concept of exchange in preference to cooperation. Noting the powerful social value attached to cooperation, especially
in the health and welfare realm, they say,

> Instead of considering "good will" among agencies and the
> personalities and affability of individual executives, how-
> ever important these may be, our attention is directed to the
> organizational factors that affect the flow of specific and
> measurable elements (i.e., patients, personnel, and nonhuman
> resources) which are the life-blood of organizational activ-
> ity and maintenance. Accordingly, the student of health and
> welfare agencies must not take at face value generic comments
> about the desirability of greater coordination and coopera-
> tion but must ascertain (1) the problems of health and wel-
> fare agencies, (2) the specific types of cooperation sought,
> (3) of whom, and (4) for whom.

The conditions under which exchange may occur have been
examined by a number of writers who have considered intergroup networks. J. Kenneth Benson (1975) considers the problem of *work
coordination* among organizations, which is similar to the concept
of interorganizational exchange. "Work is coordinated to the extent that programs and activities in two or more organizations are
geared into each other with a maximum of effectiveness and efficiency."

High work coordination among organizations tends to be related to high:

• *Positive evaluation*--the judgment by workers in one organization of the value of the work of another organization,

• *Ideological consensus*--agreement among participants in organizations regarding the nature of the tasks confronted by the
organizations and the appropriate approaches to those tasks, and

• *Domain consensus*--agreement among participants in organizations regarding the appropriate role and scope of an agency.

To illustrate these concepts, one would not expect high
levels of resource flow (exchange) between health units that did
not make a high *positive evaluation* of each other's work. This is
essentially a matter of perceived competency. Although osteopaths
and medical doctors now share the same philosophy of healing, the
latter may evaluate the work of the former as inferior, which
would hamper exchange relationships. The quality of individual
units as well as categories of services are open to evaluation.
So a physician, a clinic, or a hospital judged to provide sub-
standard health services may be excluded from the exchange network.

The concept of *ideological consensus* seems especially pertinent in identifying units that would not be expected to interrelate with each other. One would not expect a Catholic hospital and an abortion clinic to enter exchange relationships, nor a laetrile practitioner and a comprehensive cancer center oncologist, nor a Christian Science reader and a psychiatrist. In each, the principal interference to possible exchange would be ideological. In reality there may be some exchange among practitioners or other health service units with low ideological consensus. For example, folk practitioners and medical doctors may relate to each other and develop mutual respect under certain conditions, and a certain amount of referral may take place between chiropractors and medical doctors.

Domain consensus is a term often used in tandem with *exchange* in explaining the ordering of independent groups. While specialized groups may engage in exchange relationships for their mutual benefit, there may be competition and conflict among them, especially for those groups that offer the same or substitutable services. A means of maintaining order in potential conflict situations is to establish agreement among groups on their respective domains--domain consensus. Referring specifically to health organizations, Levine and White (1961) say,

> . . . there can be no exchange of elements without some agreement or understanding, however implicit. These exchange agreements are contingent upon the organization's domain. . . . In operational terms, organizational domain in the health field refers to the claims that an organization stakes out for itself in terms of (1) disease covered, (2) population served, and (3) services rendered. . . . Exchange agreements rest upon prior consensus regarding domain. Within the health agency systems, consensus regarding an organization's domain must exist to the extent that parts of the system will provide each agency with the elements necessary to attain its ends.

The attempt to establish clear distinctions between primary, secondary, and tertiary services is an exercise in establishing domain consensus in the services rendered. The reluctance of family physicians to refer patients to specialists, which sometimes occurs, may result from fear that the patient will not be returned (that the specialist will impinge upon the domain of primary practice). Categorization of emergency medical services by level of service discussed earlier is an effort at defining domain. Geoffrey Gibson's comment that the reactions of most community hospitals to such categorization has been "hostile, deeply felt and successful" demonstrates that establishing domain is not automatic nor always achieved (Gibson, 1977). Thus domain is likely to be an accommodation to intergroup competition and conflict and open to challenge in the dynamics of interorganizational relationships.

Mediated Fields

In a mediated field a mechanism is introduced to coordinate activities of units in the field. As pointed out earlier, a distinction is made by Lehman between mediating mechanisms and guiding mechanisms. This is a distinction in the location of control. In a mediated field, control remains with the member group whereas guided fields rely on control from a single source. A prototype of mediating mechanisms is the health and hospital councils found in many cities and regions.

Basil Mott (1971) has written in detail on this type of interorganizational field. He identifies types of fields that are parallel to Lehman's. His first division is between unmanaged coordination (feudal) and managed coordination (mediated field, guided field) and then he divides managed coordination between peer coordination (mediated field) and hierarchical coordination (guided field). Mott's work focuses on coordination by peer councils--thus on mediated coordination. His conclusions are based on a detailed analysis of the Interdepartmental Health and Hospital Council (IHHC) of New York State. IHHC was a mechanism established by the governor of New York and thus had greater resources and legitimacy than many such councils. Mott, however, concluded that the IHHC was an ineffective organizational mechanism for making decisions. "As a decision-making body, the Council did little more than make it easier for members to reach agreements and increase somewhat the likelihood that the objectives agreed upon would be achieved" (Mott, 1968). In a generalizing statement, drawing a distinction between coordinating councils and hierarchical organizations, Mott says,

> Coordinating councils possess much poorer means of controlling member behavior. They lack formal authority over members and usually lack customary resources--funds, manpower, and prestige. . . . The control that coordinating councils have over their members is limited largely to the benefits that members derive from voluntarily cooperating with each other. Such sanctions as they may be said to possess are the benefits that members may lose by failing to cooperate and the ill will that any member may incur as a result of being uncooperative. Consequently, a coordinating council can act, on its own, and thus coordinate, only on matters on which members can agree voluntarily [Mott, 1968].

The major purpose of mediating agencies is to bring order among units that potentially are in competition or conflict. Member groups, however, do not lose their identity and for the most part seek to promote their own goals through such agencies. To a considerable extent, coordinating activities establish and preserve the domain of member groups; as such, they represent an institutionalization of domain relationships (Litwak and Hylton, 1962). Thus a motive for a hospital participating in a hospital consortium may be to protect its self-interest (domain) relative

to other hospitals. It is not uncommon for coordinating agencies
to act in order to preserve the status quo among members and to
protect them from interlopers.

Guided Fields

In a guided field, control is exercised by an agency or
administrative unit acting for the system as a whole (Lehman,
1975). This type of organization, according to Alford, is the
main challenge to the pluralism of the dominant professional
monopolists. It is also included in Mott's hierarchical coordination. At the extreme, the interorganizational field becomes a
corporate entity. Lehman considers two subtypes of guided
fields—empires and corporate fields.

Empires. In health empires a single unit becomes dominant in its
relationships with other units in the field and exercises control
over the entire field. A dominant unit may emerge from interactions within an unmanaged field, but Lehman (1975) suggests that
all relationships of asymmetrical power among units in an interorganizational field should not be regarded as health empires.
The term "health empire" is used extensively by the Health Policy
Advisory Center (Health-PAC), a community action group (in
Alford's terminology, a spokesman for *repressed structural interests*). Health-PAC's analysis of health empires in New York City,
although used as a political weapon, is nonetheless insightful.
According to Health-PAC, medical care in New York City is dominated by seven medical empires that control more than three-
quarters of the hospital beds, more than half of the health professional resources, and a lion's share of public money for biomedical and sociomedical research and development (Ehrenreich and
Ehrenreich, 1971). The cores of the empires are university
affiliated medical centers, each of which dominates a set of private and public hospitals and other health facilities in its
imperial orbit.

> Imperial power has not simply accrued, step by step, with the
> flow of public funds to the medical centers. Underlying the
> empires' growth is an internal dynamic which leads to out-
> ward expansion, usually into ghetto areas, and to concentra-
> tion of brains, facilities, money, and power at the center's
> core [Ehrenreich and Ehrenreich, 1971].

Using the same approach, Dorothy Nelkin and David Edelman
examined the centralization of resources and control in one of New
York City's medical empires, with Montefiore Hospital and Medical
Center at its core. The authors consider the following imperatives of scientific medicine:

- A hospital must have a large and stable financial base.
- Hospitals must secure a steady flow of patients to maintain
maximum utilization of their technical facilities (medical teams

can work together effectively only with regular, practical experience). Thus each hospital must be able to draw on a large population of potential clients.
  • The high costs of scientific medicine have fostered a management style in which economic efficiency must be a primary goal. "The economics of efficient management often dominate social goals, and priorities for health service programs may follow less from social need than from income produced" (Nelkin and Edelman, 1976).

In the case developed by Nelkin and Edelman, Montefiore Hospital and Medical Center was subject to these technical imperatives of scientific medicine.

> Complex techniques such as open heart surgery require a highly coordinated team of about seventeen doctors and technicians; effective teamwork can be achieved only through the experience acquired by working together on a regular basis. A high rate of utilization is also necessary for the economic viability of costly technical facilities, and this viability requires a large population base from which patients will come to Montefiore and use its special services in preference to those of other hospitals.

Such imperatives led to the West Bronx Health Planning Study, which would have closed a hospital in the area and built a new facility, North Central Bronx (NCB), adjacent to Montefiore. The authors see regionalization in this case leading to centralization, and bureaucratic-technocratic domination by a core institution—a move that was strongly resisted by community members and other health institutions in the area.
Regionalization is a rational approach to allocation of resources and organizing the health care system of an area.

> Yet with all the sensible premises embodied in the concept of regional health care, no comprehensive system exists in the United States which even approximates the idea. The reasons behind this apparent paradox are to be found in the political dimensions of regionalization plans and their anticipated effect on existing organizations and on the distribution of health care. The NCB-Montefiore case suggests that competing medical interests perceive highly rational regionalization plans simply as rationalizations for the expansion and development of medical empires [Nelkin and Edelman, 1976].

While most examples and analyses of health empires come from metropolitan areas, when considering the rural components of the health field the image of a metropolitan core with hinterland colonies seems apt. The distance from the core institution tends to reduce control of the outlying units so that rural units in

empires may retain a good deal of autonomy even if by virtue of
neglect.

The term "satellite" applies to health units as well as political units within an empire. The satellite health unit is common in rural areas and tends to be established to increase the
catchment area of a core unit and provide a source of patients for
the center.

Corporate guidance of medical care fields. A corporate field is
one in which activities of several medical care units are administered by a professional administrative unit. For example, the
Kaiser Foundation Health Plan is the central governing body of the
Kaiser-Permanente Medical Care Programs. Corporate-guided medical
care fields differ from empires in that the administrative center
is separate from any particular unit. Supposedly, decisions are
made on the basis of what is best for the field rather than for
the core unit.

Corporate guidance places managers at the center of the
medical care delivery system. "The corporate rationalist perspective implicitly assumes that health delivery systems will improve
once efficient administrative superstructures are developed and,
hence, that the delivery problem is most effectively tackled from
the top down, that is, by first rationalizing the bureaucratic
shell in which networks of health care units are nested" (Lehman,
1975). In such a field, the administrator-planner becomes the
dominant actor, and bureaucratic control, the organizational mode.
The recognition of problems such as inequity in availability of
health services, fragmentation, overlaps and gaps in health services, and need for accountability in government financial programs
upens the system to management. Cost containment, categorization
of emergency services, channeling of patients, manpower allocation, and efforts to control external environments through planning are characteristic concerns of corporate guidance.

Regionalization is a prime concept in the corporate-guidance
lexicon. Virtually every federal program that enters the medical
care delivery field stresses regionalization; Ruth Roemer et al.
(1975) say, "The essence of all rational delivery systems is
regionalization."

Some of the forms that corporate guidance takes are hospital
chains, comprehensive prepaid group practices (for example, Kaiser-
Permanente), and national health planning mechanisms.

Rural areas are especially subject to the intervention of
managers and planners. Challenges to dominant patterns come where
those patterns break down. The delivery of health services in rural areas has been a persistent problem so it is natural that conscious intervention to solve problems in rural areas be attempted.

In the following chapters unmanaged and managed interorganizational fields are the main divisions (Table 5.1). The unmanaged
field is similar to Alford's market model and Lehman's feudal
field and is informed by Levine's and White's discussion of orga-

Table 5.1. Correspondence of concepts of control in interorganizational fields

Basil Mott	Edward Lehman	Robert Alford	David Pearson	Sol Levine and Paul White
Unmanaged field	Laterally linked fields (market model, feudalism)	Professional monopolists (pluralist model)	...	Exchange
Managed field (peer group control)	Mediated field	...	Voluntary planning	...
Managed field (hierarchical control)	Guided field Empires Corporate guidance	Corporate rationalists (bureaucratic model)	Direct patient care	...

nizational exchange. The managed field is more finely divided. The discussion will utilize Lehman's distinctions within the managed field of mediated field (similar to Mott's peer group control and Pearson's voluntary planning) and guided field (similar to Mott's hierarchical control, Alford's corporate control, and Pearson's direct patient case model), which Lehman further divides into empires and corporate-guided fields.

Within the unmanaged/managed division, discussions are in terms of the three principal elements of regionalization, namely specialization or differentiation of services, spatially ordered distribution of services, and organizational control of services.

Unmanaged Regionalization
of Health Services

Since regionalization is visible in the action programs of
organized groups, whether they are government, professional, or
educational, it is almost always perceived as planned and implemented by formal agreements, including formal sanctions as means
of control. But perhaps regionalization also develops without
planning. The test is whether there is evidence of regionalization in the American health care system which has developed
largely without conscious planning and overall formal control.
This is not to contend that control is not present in the health
care field, but that it has traditionally been controlled by the
marketplace and professional relations. Independent practitioners and freestanding hospitals represent major components in
the health care system of the United States. "Entrepreneurship"
and "cottage industry" are favorite descriptions, especially by
critics, of physicians and this mode of practice. And while the
health professions are powerfully organized, their stance has
been freedom from regulation outside the profession as a means of
protecting professional autonomy.

In the preceding discussion, all the accounts of regionalization involved (1) differentiation of service on the basis of level
of service such as primary, secondary, and tertiary levels; (2)
spatial ordering of services; and (3) coordination of the differentiated services in order to provide comprehensive services to a
clientele. In this chapter and those that follow, evidence of
these characteristics in the health care system will be examined.
The argument is that to the extent that characteristics of regionalization exist on a broad level, unmanaged regionalization
exists.

DIFFERENTIATION OF UNMANAGED SERVICES

Physicians are the focal participants in the delivery of
health services. The differentiation of their services will be
considered first, followed by differentiation of hospital services.

Differentiation of Physicians' Services

At an earlier time physicians tended to be functionally simi-
lar--more or less competent as general practitioners in the art of
medicine. If divisions occurred, they were likely to be on the
basis of philosophy of healing. At the turn of the century, the
two leading schools of healing were allopathy and homeopathy, with
osteopathy and chiropractic just emerging. Differentiation of
services then was based on ideological and spatial concerns. Under these circumstances, every doctor was in competition with
every other doctor because they claimed competency in general
practice.

For practical purposes, there is now a single philosophy of
healing presented in colleges of medicine. Homeopathy has with-
ered away, osteopathy has entered the mainstream of medicine, and
chiropractic remains far on the fringe.

Today physicians are not functionally equivalent. Numerous
specialties have developed because of the vast knowledge available
in the medical sciences, the explosion in technology, and more
discriminating demands of clients. There are 22 specialties in
the medical profession offering board certification, but differentiation is much more detailed than that with much specialization
within most of the specialty designations. Specialization is not
based on differences in the philosophy of healing. It occurs
within a profession unified by professional norms that guide the
relationships among physicians of different specialties. Thus
family practitioners are specialists who find their niche at the
base of the medical care delivery system. Their special province
is the treatment of more common conditions with the expectation
that more complicated ailments will be referred to an appropriate
specialist.

The levels of medical care are commonly divided into primary, secondary, and tertiary services. Primary care represents
the entry point to the health care system. General and family
practice physicians are the clearest examples of primary care
physicians, but specialists in internal medicine, pediatrics, and
obstetrics-gynecology are often regarded as primary care physicians. Secondary services are more specialized and theoretically
obtained on the basis of referral from primary care physicians.
Most surgical procedures are performed at the secondary level,
which often involves hospitalization in community hospitals. Tertiary level services suggest the superspecialists. Such services
are not confined to any specialty designation, but one thinks of
thoracic surgeons, pediatric cardiologists, and neurosurgeons as
examples. While the three-level designation of services is widely
used, there are in fact no clear dividing points among them. A
more accurate characterization would be continua of specialization
and the realization that a given physician may provide services at
more than one level.

There has been considerable concern that general practitioners, exemplifying primary care physicians, have declined drasti-
cally in numbers. The seriousness of this problem is abated some-

what by the fact that primary care is provided by other specialists. Also, physicians are induced to enter primary care practice
through federal support of residency programs that emphasize
family practice and other primary care specialties.

Health services are provided in centers of commerce and
service--the villages, towns, and cities that dot the landscape.
Differentiation of services can be observed within the context of
service centers. Some centers obviously have very simple services, others have very complex ones, with a range of complexity
for others between these extremes. The size of the center is a
fairly good index of its complexity of services, but a more direct
index can provide more details about the characteristics of the
services and their interrelationships (Young and Young, 1973). A
technique that is quite effective in portraying the complexity of
services in the community is based on scalogram analysis developed
by Louis Guttman and commonly referred to as a Guttman scale. Although originally applied to sociopsychological data, the technique has proved useful in a wide variety of other situations including the scaling of entire societies (Udy, 1958) and communities in a wide variety of settings (Hassinger, 1957; Fuguitt and
Deeley, 1966; Young and Young, 1973). A valuable characteristic
of such scales is that there is a unique combination of responses
for each scale score (Bailey, 1978). The Guttman-type scale is
cumulative in that the combination of responses required to make a
particular score has all the responses of the next lower score,
plus one additional response category. If the items of the scale
cumulate in this manner, the scale is said to have the quality of
unidimensionality--that is, it represents an underlying single
dimension, for example, the dimension of complexity of services.
A common criterion for assessing the quality of the Guttman scale
is the coefficient of reproducibility (C.R.), which measures the
ability to reconstruct the original responses from the scale
scores or, in other words, the extent to which the scale is unidimensional. Thus if the C.R. is 0.90, there are 10 errors in a
pattern of 100 response units. A C.R. of 0.90 or 0.95 is often
used as a criterion for a high-quality scale.

An early use of the Guttman technique for analysis of community complexity was in scales of retail services, developed for
nonmetropolitan trade centers in southern Minnesota (Table 6.1).
Retail services were scaled in the following order: grocery or
general store, hardware or implement store, drug store, furniture
store, clothing store, variety store, and florist or greenhouse.
The coefficient of reproducibility was 0.98 in both 1939 and 1951
for the trade centers examined (Hassinger, 1957). Thus some centers had only very simple retail services (i.e., grocery store)
while others had more complex services (i.e., florist shop). If a
center had a florist shop, it should be noted, it would also very
likely have all the other services listed above. The success of
the scales indicates that there was (and presumably is) a regularity in the pattern of retail services in trade centers that can be
predicted with a high degree of accuracy from the scale score of a

Table 6.1. Retail service patterns of incorporated places in 43 southern Minnesota counties, 1939 and 1951

| Scale score | Distribution of incorporated places by service patterns | | | | Presence or absence of specified services or stores | | | | | | |
| | 1939 | | 1951 | | Grocery or general | Hardware or implement | Drug | Furniture | Clothing | Variety | Florist or greenhouse |
	Frequency*	Percent	Frequency+	Percent							
1	13	3.7	18	5.2	X	...	...	...	...	...	...
2	104	29.6	115	33.3	X	X	...	...	...	...	...
3	49	14.0	25	7.3	X	...	X	...	...	...	...
3	1	0.3	0	...	X	...	X	...	...	...	...
4	40	11.4	31	9.0	X	X	X	X	...	...	...
4	8	2.3	9	2.6	X	X	X	X	...	...	...
5	22	6.3	15	4.4	X	X	...	X	X	...	...
5	2	0.6	0	...	X	X	X	X	X	...	...
5	2	0.6	6	1.7	X	X	X	X	X	...	...
5	1	0.3	0	...	X	X	X	...	X	...	...
6	56	16.0	57	16.5	X	X	X	X	X	X	...
6	0	...	1	0.3	X	X	...	X	X	X	...
6	1	0.3	2	0.6	X	X	X	X	X	X	...
6	11	3.1	8	2.3	X	X	X	...	X	X	...
6	2	0.6	6	1.7	X	X	X	X	...	X	...
6	2	0.6	0	...	X	X	X	...	...	X	...
6	1	0.3	3	0.9	X	X	...	X	...	X	...
7	33	9.4	48	13.9	X	X	X	X	X	X	X
7	1	0.3	0	...	X	X	X	X	...	X	X
7	1	0.3	1	0.3	X	X	X	X	X	...	X
Total	350	100.0	345	100.0							

Source: Hassinger, 1957, p. 237. (Reprinted by permission of *Rural Sociology*)
Note: The coefficient of reproducibility was 0.98 in 1939 and 0.98 in 1951. X = presence; ... = absence.
*Incomplete data for one place.
+Incomplete data for six places.

trade center. In Table 6.1, it can be observed that some errors
in the pattern do exist, but the frequency of the centers having
error types are quite small.

Sociologists at Cornell University have utilized differentiation (and complexity) of services as a major structural variable in their community research. In a study of 144 New York
State communities ranging in size from under 1,000 population to
over 600,000, several Guttman scales were constructed, including
a retail trade scale, a community facilities scale, a housing
scale, a scale of community planning structure, and a medical
specialties scale.

Table 6.2 illustrates the characteristics of the retail service scale. Scales of this type are quite descriptive and lend
themselves to interpretation. "If the institution [service] is
specialized, it will fit into a community that has an equal or
higher level of structural differentiation than that of the institution [service] itself. Specifically, an establishment like a
bank can locate in a community only where other supporting institutions such as modern transportation and communication, real
estate office, legal services, and police already exist. . . .
What determines the bank's location in a community is the institutional base" (Moore et al., 1974). The specific errors in a pattern of services for trade centers can also reveal characteristics
of service relationships. "There is some evidence that scale
errors are 'made up' over time. If a community is lacking a particular facility, which according to the overall pattern it should
have, it is very likely to acquire that facility in the next two
years" (Taietz, 1973). It should be added that services to the
right (more complex) of the error may be vulnerable to loss from
a community. In other words, a community that is losing services
tends to, but does not always, lose them in the order of their
complexity.

If we were to apply the Guttman technique (and reasoning) to

Table 6.2. Retail trade scale

Scale score	Item	Percent of communities with scale score	Cumulative percent
0	None	0.8	0.8
1	Gas station	15.0	15.8
2	Radio, TV, music	6.0	21.8
3	Family shoe store	7.5	29.3
4	Retail bakery	10.5	39.8
5	Book and stationery	6.0	45.8
6	Reupholstery	9.7	55.5
7	Department store	10.5	66.0
8	Millinery and hosiery	9.8	75.8
9	Furrier	6.8	82.6
10	Egg and poultry	6.8	89.4
11	Auto service	6.8	96.2
12	Parking	3.8	100.0

Source: Taietz, 1973.
Note: C.R. = 0.95.

Table 6.3. Hypothetical physician services pattern

Scale types (score)	Number communities* (over 1,000 pop.)	Physician services		
		Primary	Secondary	Tertiary
1	25	0	0	0
2	100	+	0	0
3	25	+	+	0
4	10	+	+	+

Note: + = presence; 0 = absence.
*Hypothetical.

physician services in communities and utilize the primary, secondary, and tertiary distinction in health services made earlier, we
might guess that some places would have no medical services, some
only primary services, some secondary services (but we would guess
that those with secondary services would also have primary services), and some would have tertiary services (but we would guess
that those places would also have secondary and primary services)
(Table 6.3). If types of physician services are scaled in this
manner without error, one could predict the exact pattern of services by knowing the scale score. A score of 2, for example, would
mean the presence of a primary care physician in the community,
but not a secondary or tertiary physician. A score of 4 would assure the observer that a community had not only tertiary services
but also secondary and primary medical services.

Of direct interest is the medical specialties scale developed
for New York communities (Table 6.4). The C.R. of 0.96 indicates
that a highly regular cumulative pattern exists. The content of
the scale also conforms well to expectations on the basis of primary, secondary, and tertiary health services. The foundation
(and most numerous) of physician services is primary care, which
is found in general practice, general surgery, internal medicine,

Table 6.4. Medical specialties scale

Scale score	Item	Percent of communities with scale score	Cumulative percent
0	None	0.7	0.7
1	General practitioner	19.2	19.9
2	General surgeon	12.4	32.3
3	Internal medicine	10.9	43.2
4	Obstetrician-gynecologist	10.9	54.1
5	Pediatrician	3.7	57.8
6	Radiologist	2.2	60.0
7	Ophthalmologist	3.7	63.7
8	Pathologist	5.2	68.9
9	Otolaryngologist	7.4	76.3
10	Urologist	10.9	87.2
11	Allergist	4.4	91.6
12	Colon and rectal surgeon	2.3	93.9
13	Plastic surgeon	1.5	95.4
14	Neurologist	1.5	96.9
15	Child psychiatrist	2.4	99.3
16	Pediatric cardiologist	0.7	100.0

Source: Taietz, 1973.
Note: C.R. = 0.96.

obstetrics-gynecology, and pediatrics. There probably would be
general agreement at the other end of the scale that plastic surgeons, neurologists, child psychiatrists, and pediatric cardiologists are highly specialized practitioners and are often associated with tertiary level care. Note also that less than 6 percent
of the communities have any of these five specialties.

In a manner similar to the previous research, John Foley
produced a Guttman scale of local health care differentiation,
which is an 18-item scale measuring the presence in a community
(county) of a variety of AMA board certified physicians (Table
6.5). The data are from 274 counties in 12 eastern states. The
scale reaches a higher level of complexity (items of greater specialization are included) than was true for the New York communities cited previously. But, as with the New York communities, the

Table 6.5. Guttman scale of local health care differentiation

Order of items	Frequency	Errors
18 Hematology	2	3
17 Clinical microbiology	5	3
16 Radium therapy	9	5
15 Pediatric cardiology	14	7
14 Psychiatry and neurology	16	12
13 Allergy	22	4
12 Therapeutic radiology	26	13
11 Colon and rectal surgery	34	6
10 Physical medicine and rehabilitation	48	13
9 Plastic surgery	61	10
8 Neurological surgery	79	10
7 Dermatology and syphilology	107	17
6 Orthopedic surgery	135	10
5 Urology	146	19
4 Obstetrics and gynecology	166	15
3 Ophthalmology	181	20
2 Radiology	205	18
1 Surgery	236	5

Source: John W. Foley, Community structure and the de-
terminants of local health care differentiation. *Social
Forces* 56(Dec. 1977):655. (Reprinted by permission of The
University of North Carolina Press)
Note: C.R. = 0.96; n = 274.

patterning is present with considerable regularity--C.R. of 0.96.
Foley, in assessing the implication of the pattern for social
change, notes: "Local health differentiation seems to proceed in
a stepwise progression. In attempting to attract health care
specialists the most reasonable goal would be to either 'fill-in'
the scale by attracting specialists who were not present but
'should have been' (so called 'errors') according to the community's position on the scale or by seeking to attract to the community a physician who practices the medical specialty one step
above the highest level now present" (Foley, 1977).

Differentiation of Hospitals

Service differentiation is also characteristic of hospitals.
Aside from the existence of specialty hospitals dealing with cancer, tuberculosis, and mental illness, short-term general hospi-

tals offer quite different levels of service. The range is from large medical centers with beds numbered in the thousands to small hospitals in rural communities with fewer than 25 beds. Ralph Berry, in a study of short-term general hospitals, found that there was a definite and systematic pattern to the expansion of services in such institutions. Berry (1973) says, "There is such a thing as a basic service hospital. As hospitals add facilities and services, there is a strong tendency to first add those that enhance the *quality* of basic services. Only after the services that enhance the quality of the basic services have been acquired do short-term general hospitals display a tendency to expand the complexity of the scope of services provided. The final stage of expansion process for certain hospitals occurs when they add facilities and services that essentially transform them from inpatient institutions to community medical centers." Berry does not use the scaling terminology or tests of scalability associated with Guttman scales, but it is apparent that the four types of hospitals and their services could be treated in the following manner:

(1) Basic--clinical laboratory, emergency room, operating room, delivery room, diagnostic X ray;

(2) Quality enhancing--blood bank, pathology laboratory, pharmacy and pharmacist, premature nursery, postoperative recovery room;

(3) Complex--electroencephalography, dental facilities, physical therapy, intensive care units, therapeutic X ray, radioisotope therapy, psychiatric inpatient units, cobalt therapy, radium therapy;

(4) Community--occupational therapy, outpatient department, home care program, social work department, rehabilitation unit, family planning service.

Berry found that in the United States basic hospitals were most numerous and community hospitals least numerous. The average size of each type of hospital was about double the type below it, with basic hospitals averaging 43 beds and community hospitals 450. The bed occupancy ratio was 65 percent for basic type hospitals and over 80 percent for community type hospitals.

Differentiation of hospitals can also be noted in the categorization of scope of capabilities for providing emergency medical services. The range is from only limited to comprehensive and highly sophisticated emergency services. The criteria for categorizing the emergency service capabilities of hospitals are given in Chapter Four.

In addition, it was found in a national sample of 480 hospitals that implementation of five programs (home care services, family planning, medical social work, mental health, and rehabilitation) was taken in the step-by-step manner judged to be unidimensional by the Guttman scaling criterion (C.R. = 0.91) (Kaluzny et al., 1971). It is pertinent to note that these distinctions

among hospitals exist not on the basis of conscious planning but
because of the forces of the marketplace and entrepreneurship.

SPATIAL ORDERING OF UNMANAGED SERVICES
     The differentiation of health services which was observed
implies that there will be order in the geographical distribution
of the services. Spatial ordering will be examined, broadly utilizing the rural/urban, metropolitan/nonmetropolitan distinction
and at a finer level dealing with the areal relations among service centers for which the concept of regionalization is most
pertinent.

Metropolitan/Nonmetropolitan Distribution
     It is not news that rural areas have deficient physician/pop-
ulation ratios when compared with urban areas. The ratio is more
than twice as great for metropolitan as for nonmetropolitan areas.
Furthermore, the ratio in the most rural counties is less than
one-fourth that of metropolitan counties. As one examines the
data in Table 6.6, it can be seen that the metropolitan/nonmetro-
politan, urban/rural differences are accounted for by the differences in relative numbers of specialists in the respective areas.
General practitioner/population ratios are quite uniform for all
population categories. The specialist/metropolitan population
ratios, however, far exceed those in the nonmetropolitan categories. It is also of interest to note that there are not sharp
differences in subcategories of metropolitan/nonmetropolitan,
specialist/population ratios but rather a gradual shift from the
more metropolitan categories through the more rural categories.
Those nonmetropolitan counties having an urban population of
20,000 or more (classified in the table as nonmetropolitan, urbanized) are much more likely than more rural counties to have specialists in residence. Many places of this size serve as service
centers for a wide rural area and have quite sophisticated health
facilities and personnel. It appears, then, that even in those
rural communities where physicians are present, individuals must
look to larger centers for more specialized medical services.
Thus in aggregate, there is a dependence by rural populations on
urban areas for comprehensive health services.

Ordering of Central Places
     There has been a great deal of interest by social scientists
in the location patterns of market centers. The problem has
gained the attention of economists, geographers, anthropologists,
and sociologists. The work of Walter Christaller (1933/1966), a
geographer, developed a theoretical basis for the location of market centers of different service complexity. Christaller sought
to determine the optimal location of retail firms based on marketing principles given the assumptions of an even distribution of
population and purchasing power, unvarying physical landscape, and

Table 6.6. Physicians in patient care per 100,000 population by type of practice and residence, 1975

Residence	General practitioners	Office-based			Hospital-based
		Medical specialists	Surgical specialists	Other specialists	
		(number per 100,000 population)			
Metropolitan	19.9	30.9	36.3	25.6	44.7
Greater	20.4	35.5	37.7	29.0	55.1
Core	21.7	39.3	41.9	32.2	68.9
Fringe	17.4	27.0	28.4	21.8	24.4
Medium	19.5	25.4	34.3	21.3	33.6
Lesser	18.7	24.1	34.7	21.6	26.2
Nonmetropolitan	25.9	10.5	18.3	9.2	7.4
Urbanized					
Adjacent	22.9	15.5	25.7	13.0	10.3
Nonadjacent	21.6	19.7	33.9	17.7	14.2
Less urbanized					
Adjacent	27.7	6.6	11.6	5.6	6.1
Nonadjacent	29.9	7.7	15.2	7.4	4.5
Totally rural					
Adjacent	25.3	1.7	3.5	1.8	2.5
Nonadjacent	26.1	2.9	4.5	2.7	1.8
U.S. total	21.5	25.3	31.4	21.2	34.6

Source: Ahearn, 1979.

uniform transportation system in all directions, so that all central places of the same type were equally accessible. The model
is based on the reasoning that all parts of the region should be
supplied with all conceivable goods from the fewest possible central places. It is of interest, for our present discussion, that
Christaller's favorite example was the provision of physicians'
services. However, from the context of the discussion, it is
clear that he was thinking of the general physician, not the
specialist.

Christaller's presentation was detailed and technical. The
following is a concise statement by Carol A. Smith (1976) in her
introduction of a series of papers by anthropologists on regional
analysis.

> Christaller approached the problem by considering the amount
> of business a retail firm could expect to get from distant
> consumers--the *range* of the good or service provided. He
> defined the range of a good as the circular area beyond
> which buyers would not be willing to travel for the good,
> given need (elasticity of demand), price, transportation
> cost (which is added to price), and frequency of use. . . .
> Christaller also had to consider the supplier and the amount
> of business he needs to stay in business--his economic
> *threshold*. This threshold was defined as the circular area
> containing sufficient consumer demand of a good to meet the
> supplier's requirements for survival in business.
>   . . . From these two principles (and using the example
> of physicians), one can model consumer and supplier behavior
> in interaction with each other. That is, given consumer den-
> sity, needs, and income (which add up to demand), and given
> supplier price and income requirements (which add up to
> ability to supply), plus knowledge of transport costs, one
> should be able to predict how many physicians a given area
> can support, the actual physical area that would meet the
> physician's threshold. From all of that, one could estimate
> the appropriate--most economic--spacing of physicians on the
> landscape. While such a prediction would be quite a feat,
> Christaller was even more ambitious. He wanted to explain
> the distribution of *all* retail firms in a region, from gro-
> cery stores to physicians, to rare book stores. His model,
> therefore, basically attends to various *levels* of centers
> (central places) and their distributions--to the special pat-
> terns of central-place *systems*.

This can be applied to different levels of health services resulting from specialization of personnel and facilities (i.e., primary, secondary, and tertiary).

> Central-place systems can be built from the top down or from
> the bottom up; Christaller worked from the top down. He
> began with suppliers of a high-order good (one for which

demand is so low or infrequent that it requires many consumers), assuming that as many suppliers as possible attempt to locate in a region to saturate all demand, and uncovered an optimal locational pattern for them, as follows. Each supplier will attempt to locate as far as possible from the other suppliers in order to dominate as many consumers as possible; thus, each supplier begins with a circular demand area. But when the numerous suppliers saturate a region up to their absolute minimum thresholds, the circles will overlap. Packing of circles (from competition), and consumer choice of the closest supplier with the lowest price (consumer rationality), will bisect the areas of overlap, ultimately leading to hexagonal market areas for each supplier, as well as to the minimum supplier price. Both supplier threshold and consumer range will be minimized. (It should be noted that this process assumes maximizing behavior by both supplier and consumer as well as perfect competition.)

Then Christaller took suppliers of a lower-order good (one for which demand is more frequent) and attempted to place them on the same landscape. He assumed that these suppliers would also be in competition and would choose locations in terms of greatest advantage, as follows. They would first locate in the centers that provided higher-order goods (first-level centers), thus inveigling business that was attracted to the higher-order goods. But since demand for the goods of this second group was sufficient to give them a lower threshold than the first suppliers, they would next locate at the interstices between the packed higher-order suppliers, thereby meeting the greatest possible demand and the least possible competition. This would provide second-level centers between first-level centers. The process would be the same for suppliers of a third order and of lower orders of goods that would produce even lower-level centers between first- and second-level centers, and then between second- and third-level centers, and so on.

The consequences of this particular locational process are as follows: The high-level centers would become larger and more widely spaced than lower-level centers. All higher level centers would supply both high- and low-order goods, and low-level centers would provide only low-order goods and nest in the trade areas of high-level centers. . . . From the point of view of the consumer, who is providing the demand that influences supplier decisions about location, this pattern has many advantages. It provides many small centers that carry items needed frequently, so that no consumer is very far from one of them. It also provides larger centers that carry items of less frequent demand together with items needed more often, so that on the rare occasion that one might need a funeral parlor, say, one could also buy the weekly groceries and thus spread transport costs over the several items. Finally it provides for competitive pricing

by suppliers. Should any supplier charge a much higher fee
than another, he would lose the customer at the boundaries
of his hinterland, because the most distant consumers in his
"natural" trade area could afford the extra transport cost of
utilizing another supplier with the savings from a lower
price. Hence, suppliers should stabilize close to their mar-
gins, the distant consumer disciplining what would otherwise
be the topological monopoly of each supplier [Smith, 1976].

On the basis of the preceding reasoning, a system of central
places was postulated as shown in Figure 6.1. This well-known
figure shows the arrangement of centers offering different levels
of services. Each lower level central place, for example, is located at the midpoint between three higher level centers.

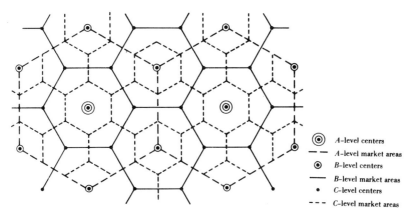

◎	A-level centers
– – –	A-level market areas
◉	B-level centers
———	B-level market areas
•	C-level centers
- - -	C-level market areas

Fig. 6.1. A hierarchical spatial arrangement of central
          places according to Christaller's k = 3 principle.
          (From Lloyd and Dicken, 1972. Reprinted by per-
          mission of Harper and Row)

The question is whether the geographical distribution of physicians and various other specialized health services approaches
a system that conforms to the marketing principles of central
place location. It is clear that Christaller's model is based on
assumptions that do not exist in the real world (i.e., uniform
transportation in all directions, homogeneous topography, uniform
distribution of population, populations of similar tastes, prefer-
ences, and income). But the question with these kinds of qualifi-
cations remains whether the theory informs us about the real
world. Such a service landscape would provide an "economically
appropriate" distribution of services whereby services would be
available in as many places as there was "economic" demand for
them. It is an important point to make that lesser order centers
would not be satellites of higher order centers; rather they

would be competitive with them on the lower order of services, and
by virtue of location at the interstices of three larger central
places their areas would be divided among higher level centers for
higher order services.

Evidence of the Effects of Marketing Principles on the Distribution of Health Services

Central place theory provides a plausible conceptualization
of the location of health care services. Different levels of
services (i.e., primary, secondary, and tertiary) are commonly
identified. Specialty services were shown in the earlier discussion of Guttman-type scales of physicians' specialties to be distributed among service centers in a cumulative manner. The geographical distribution of service centers (more complex centers at
greater intervals, simpler centers at more frequent intervals)
suggests that marketing principles are operating to some extent.
The general feeling that central place location based on marketing
principles is applicable to the health care system is supported
by Brian Berry (1967) who examined consumers' use of services for
physicians and hospitals along with other services, including retail groceries, lawyers, women's clothing stores, and daily news-
papers. He found variations in travel patterns depending on the
service used, which led him to conclude that "the process whereby
Christaller locates smaller centers relative to higher-order centers is not unlike the development process observed in Iowa."

Analysts can readily develop models of optimum location of
services using population distributions, distance, cost, and other
demand factors. William Hardy (1972), for example, has designated
a model based on economic principles for the location of rural
health outreach clinics.

Due to dissatisfaction with analyses based on physician/popu-
lation ratios for political units (mostly counties), Frank Dickinson, an economist who directed the Bureau of Medical Economic
Research of the American Medical Association, delineated primary
medical service areas for the nation. Primary medical service
areas were based on the trade area concept. According to Dickinson (1954), "A trading area is described by its centers and boundaries. A primary trading center is a town that draws considerable
trade from the surrounding territory and loses relatively little
trade to other towns. We adapted this definition of the primary
center in defining a primary medical center, as a town which,
relative to the surrounding territory, was a source of physicians'
services." Secondary medical centers (more limited services) and
prime-primary centers (most complex services) were also identified. Thus the service centers represented a hierarchical patterning. The analysis was almost entirely based on 757 primary
medical service areas, with extensive use of maps. Dickinson's
conclusion was, "The distribution of physicians in the United
States in April, 1950, in relation to the persons whom they served,
was excellent but not perfect." Areas most notably underserved
were the sparsely settled areas of western states.

In a later study modeled somewhat after Dickinson's research, it was concluded that in the upper Midwest (Minnesota, North Dakota, South Dakota, Montana) the distribution of physicians in relation to population was not seriously deficient in 1965. "Over-all the distribution of physicians followed the population distribution reasonably well. In Minnesota, where population densities are similar to the average for the United States, remarkably few people were remote from a physician by our definition (15 or more miles). In the Dakotas, with lower population densities, more people were found to be remote from a physician and in Montana, with its unusually low density, somewhat more than one in 10 of the population could be placed in the remote category" (Fahs and Peterson, 1968).

A somewhat different type of evidence of the effectiveness of the marketplace in locating services comes from an examination of the location of Emergency Medical Services (EMS) in northern California, which included an extensive rural area. Using a criterion of 13 minutes response time (the time elapsed between notification of an emergency and arrival at the emergency site), it was determined that the 15 facilities already in the area would serve 75 percent of the population. It would take 31 facilities placed optimally to get ambulance services to 86 percent of the population within the 13-minute time criterion. If the time criterion were raised to 27 minutes, 14 sites already in place could serve 95.5 percent of the population. The 15th site in the present system could be eliminated without loss of percent of coverage at this response time level, but it would take 22 sites to serve 97.7 percent of the population in an optimal location system. The conclusion of the authors was that "EMS facilities that comply with response time standards, similar to those of urban areas, were prohibitively costly in the rural parts of the study area. Increasing the response time standards reduced the regional cost of the EMS systems and allowed some of the individual EMS facilities to become economically viable, since additional people could be served by each facility" (Daberkow and King, 1977). These data also indicate that the unplanned location of EMS facilities was quite good from a cost/effect standpoint. It would take substantially more resources for a relatively small increase in the proportion of population served for a given response time.

Another set of data that bears on the question of the market principles underlying the location of health services is the problem and generally unsuccessful experience of making planned health clinics economically viable. For example, an analysis was made of economic records of six rural clinics established by the National Health Service Corps (NHSC) and staffed by midlevel practitioners (physician assistants and nurse practitioners). Four of the clinics were located in the Pacific Northwest and two in Alaska. At the end of two and one-half years, none of the practices had reached self-sufficiency. Overall, the utilization of the facilities was low, averaging between 8 and 12 patients per site per day. Moscovice and Rosenblatt (1979) point out that there is a

minimum population for attaining financial self-sufficiency in
practices of this type.

> Using generally accepted measures of utilization and fees, we
> can see that it requires a minimum population of 1,500 who
> would see the provider an average of three times a year at an
> average fee of $10 per encounter and a collection rate of
> 100 percent to generate $45,000 a year revenue. This figure
> represents a bare minimum for the support of one mid-level
> practitioner, without considering the cost of capitalizing
> facilities or equipment. Thus, it could be predicted that
> remote areas with smaller populations would be unable to sus-
> tain an independent NHSC mid-level practice without continu-
> ing subsidy.

With special reference to Alaska, the authors point out that in
extremely remote small villages, utilization is low and operating
expenses are high, and although good management and experience can
reduce costs, the major decision revolves around the question of
equity. "If we as a society decide to make curative health care
readily available to remote populations, we will have to increase
external subsidies to increasingly smaller communities" (Moscovice
and Rosenblatt, 1979).

The same authors examined 25 new rural practices in the
Pacific Northwest established by the NHSC and manned by physicians. They found that a service area population below 4,000 was
an impediment to success (Rosenblatt and Moscovice, 1978).

Health for Underserved Rural Areas (HURA) was a program that
supported demonstration projects for the delivery of primary
health services to underserved rural areas with special emphasis
on the promotion of rural health clinics. According to an HURA
staff report to the Senate Appropriations Committee, most HURA
supported projects had difficulty in achieving financial self-
sufficiency.[1] For example, during a six-month period in 1978,
collections amounted to only 40 percent of the operating cost for
health services delivered to patients. This does not take into
account the substantial capital outlay by communities and the
federal government for start-up costs. A number of clinics made
progress toward self-sufficiency, but the report noted that certain of the clinics were unlikely to achieve self-sufficiency
because of low population density or an inadequate reimbursement
system. The report indicates that many HURA projects would not
survive without continued grant support. On the basis of a detailed cost study of 29 HURA clinics it was concluded that only 5
could be expected with any confidence to maintain their current
program level without HURA funding after 1979.

----

1. The Health Underserved Rural Areas Program Status Report
as of December 31, 1978, prepared for the Senate Appropriation
Committee by the Department of Health, Education and Welfare,
Bureau of Community Health Services, Office of Rural Health.

Utilizing a central place framework specifically drawn from Walter Christaller, John Leyes and associates (1973) attempted to relate the distribution of health services to the market pattern of an area that included all of Wyoming plus parts of adjacent states. Seven levels of economic activity were identified and the seven orders of centers providing these activities were found to be hierarchical in structure (i.e., higher level centers had all the economic activities of lesser centers plus additional ones as in Guttman scales). The levels of the centers (from higher to lesser) were named (1) regional trade centers, (2) subregional trade centers, (3) wholesale/retail centers, (4) primary shopping centers, (5) secondary shopping centers, (6) convenience centers, and (7) minimum convenience centers and hamlets. Estimates were made of the service areas of level 5 centers and above, which were then plotted on a map. While there was some order in the geographical dispersion of the different levels of centers, their location and the service areas were a far cry from the neat hexagonal patterns that central place theory portrays. In a parallel manner, a hierarchy of health service centers in the area was identified and given the following names: (1) regional health care centers, (2) subregional health care centers, (3) primary health care centers, (4) secondary health care centers, (5) health care convenience centers, (6) minimum health care centers, and (7) subminimum health care centers.[2] When these types of health centers are placed on a map and the estimated health service areas are delineated around them, there is a clear correspondence between economic activity and health service patterns. Based on statistical analysis which involved 74 economic variables for the economic centers and 24 health service variables for the health centers, it was established that the correspondence between levels of economic and health centers was very high. The coefficient of multiple determination was $R^2 = 0.97$, which can be interpreted to mean that 97 percent of the variance in the levels of the health care system is explained by the economic system. The unmistakable conclusion is that there is a very close correspondence between the location of economic and health care services in the inter-mountain West, although neither system approaches the regularity in location that central place theory suggests (Leyes et al., 1973).

CONTROL IN UNMANAGED REGIONALIZATION

We can visualize a health delivery system based on specialization of services and ordered spatially according to marketplace principles. But how are the separate units coordinated in order to deliver comprehensive health services? In Chapter Five, attention was given to the control process of unmanaged fields. The process was based on exchange of resources (especially referral of

---

2. Note that primary and secondary centers reverse the conventional terminology used in health services research.

clients) to the mutual advantage of units in the field. The principal mechanism applicable to clients is professional referral in
a system in which the units are compatible in ideology, evaluate
each other as competent, and respect each other's domain.

An underlying idea of the marketplace approach is that consumers have perfect information and act in their own self-interest. Consumers of health services are offered a variety of health
services from which to choose, and by their choices become coordi-
nators of the health care system; thus services expand or contract
depending on public demand. This scenario is modified by the providers of health services through professional control, the basis
for which is that legitimacy is monopolized by the medical establishment, which is virtually without challengers in the health
care field. And within the orthodox medical establishment, physicians have achieved the apex of professional control as indicated
by their practice autonomy. The main professional alternative to
orthodox medicine, chiropractic, is a weak shadow, and osteopathy,
a potential challenger, has been completely coopted by the regular
medical profession. That leaves threats to the hegemony of physicians only from within the system. Threats are most likely to
come from administrators as organizations become more bureaucratic
or from other health professionals within the system (such as
nurses) as changes take place in the organization of the health
care system.

Professional Referral
        Nonetheless, in a profession that has become highly special-
ized and in a health care system of differentiated facilities, a
mechanism is needed to integrate the separate units. Professional
control is such a mechanism. In keeping with our explanation of
the unmanaged health delivery system, this mechanism depends on
informal understandings based on collegial relationships, which
were recognized early in the development of medical sociology by
Oswald Hall (1946) when he showed the importance of informal networks among physicians in providing order, ascribing and maintaining status, controlling conduct of members, and minimizing competition and conflict.

The professional referral system is of specific interest in
understanding the integration of units of the health care system
in providing comprehensive care. It is based on the idea that at
certain points in a patient's care a given physician is not the
most qualified person to diagnose or treat a condition and/or that
more sophisticated facilities are needed. That decision and the
choice of consultant remains a professional prerogative, and there
is considerable order in the process. The rationale for ordering
the relationship is based on entrance to the health care system
via a primary care physician and referrals to physicians practicing secondary and/or tertiary levels of medicine. Physicians at
these levels in turn are dependent on primary care physicians for
patients.

The Family-Doctor Relationship

The relationship between consumer and family doctor becomes more structured although it is still informal. This relationship takes the form of exchanges with benefits and obligations on the part of both parties. Physicians receive the benefit of a stable and known clientele; their obligation is to stand ready to provide medical care. The benefit to clients is that medical care is assured; the client's obligation is to utilize the family doctor as the initial professional contact in an illness. It is a breach of the relationship to shop around for medical care or bypass the family doctor in obtaining specialty services and most certainly to use another type of practitioner such as a chiropractor.

The family-doctor relationship is supported by the medical profession. A committee under the auspices of the American Medical Association (1966) said, "The family physician is one who . . . evaluates the patient's total health needs, provides personal medical care within one or more fields of medicine and refers the patient, when indicated, to appropriate sources of care while preserving the continuity of care." In a similar vein, a principal recommendation of the National Commission on Community Health (1966) was,

> Every individual should have a personal physician who is the central point for integration and continuity of all medical and medically related services to his patients. . . . He will either render, or direct the patient to whatever services best suit his needs. His concern will be for the patient as a whole and his relationship with the patient will be a continuing one.

The family doctor's gatekeeper role. The family-doctor relationship is not only an exchange relationship between consumer and provider but also a point of access by the patient to a complex medical care system. Physicians act as gatekeepers to the system. The gatekeeper controls access by outsiders to scarce, valued services or objects. For their part, outsiders must want the services, be unwilling to substitute others for them, and be unwilling or unable to bypass the gatekeeper in order to obtain them. Thus a gatekeeper controls access to a monopoly of goods or services.

In the abstract family-doctor relationship, monopoly of access to medical care services is clearly implied. In reality, clients have alternatives. They may bypass the family doctor and seek and often gain access to specialists directly. In addition, there are other institutionalized access points to the regular medical care system such as hospital emergency rooms, hospital outpatient clinics, and neighborhood health clinics. It is of interest that these points of contact are often referred to as family doctor substitutes. Also challenging the role of family doctor as gatekeeper are alternative types of practitioners such

as chiropractors, faith healers, and others. Nurse practitioners
and physician assistants are potential challengers of the family
doctor's gatekeeper role. To the extent that these alternatives
exist, and that people are willing to use them without referral
from the family doctor, the gatekeeper role of the family doctor
is jeopardized.

In addition, the family doctor must have at his disposal the
facilities of the medical care system if he is to effectively fulfill his role as gatekeeper. Following the decision to refer a
patient, a family doctor makes two additional judgments: the type
of specialist to which to refer the patient and the choice of a
particular specialist. Theoretically these are completely rational judgments depending on diagnosis, selection of the proper
specialty, and identifying the best-qualified practitioner. In
reality, the type of specialty depends on the diagnosis and orien-
tation of the referring physician, both of which are variable from
physician to physician. In addition, a physician's information
about practitioners in a given specialty area is limited, and
choices may be further constrained by mutual obligations between
physicians or between physician and health center (Shortell,
1973).

Furthermore, the family doctor may be reluctant to refer even
when it is beneficial to the patient, because once a patient enters the larger health care system, the family doctor may lose
control of the case and the patient. In addition, the family doctor may be poorly connected to the health care system; an example
would be an elderly doctor in a small town who has few professional contacts with other physicians.

Empirical evidence of the family-doctor relationship. In recent
literature it is more common to find the term "regular source of
medical care" than "family doctor." However, there is considerable conceptual overlap in the terms. It is clear that most persons in the United States have a regular source of medical care,
and the majority can identify a specific doctor by name--thus a
family doctor. In a survey conducted by the National Opinion
Research Center (NORC) during the year 1975-1976, using a national
representative sample of 7,787 persons, 88 percent reported they
had a regular source of medical care. Seventy-eight percent identified a doctor by name, which would be very close to the operational definition of family doctor, while 10 percent reported an
institution such as an outpatient clinic or hospital emergency
room as a regular source or that they used several doctors. Of
the 12 percent without a regular source of health care, 7 percent
indicated they were seldom ill and therefore did not need a regular doctor, 3 percent had no doctor because they had moved recently or their doctor had recently terminated his practice, and 2
percent were unable to obtain regular care (Aiken et al., 1979).
The proportion of people who report a source of regular care appears to be quite stable over a period of time. In a national
survey in 1963, 87 percent of the population had a source of reg-

ular care; 76 percent named a physician, while 11 percent named a clinic (Andersen et al., 1972).

Rural populations are not much different from urban populations in this respect. In the 1975-1976 NORC study, 93 percent of the farm residents had regular sources of medical care compared with 88 percent of the total population and 87 percent of the suburban residents. In a rural California community, 82 percent of the individuals had regular sources of medical care (Luft et al., 1976). And in Missouri, where the inquiry was specifically about a family doctor, 86 percent of the families in four rural communities reported having a family doctor compared with 81 percent in a metropolitan center in the same state (Hassinger and Hobbs, 1973).

Data indicate, however, that the family-doctor relationship may be too fragile to support the pivotal role attributed to it. Even while acknowledging such a relationship, clients may bypass the family doctor in seeking specialty services for self-diagnosed ailments. In addition, the division between doctors who render primary care, and thus are potential family doctors, and those who provide specialty care, and thus should receive patients through the referral mechanism, is not as clear-cut as the ideal would imply. Information on some 400,000 patient encounters was extracted from logs kept by a national sample of more than 10,000 physicians in 24 specialties in a study done at the University of Southern California. Patient encounters were sorted into five groups: first encounter, episodic care, principal care, consultative care, and specialized care (Table 6.7). The principal care physician appears to be closest to the concept of the family doctor. The description of principal care is as follows: "There is evidence of continuity; the physician reports having seen the patient before and considers him or her to be a regular patient. Comprehensiveness is suggested, since the physician indicates that he or she provides most of the patient's needs" (Aiken et al., 1979). The authors elaborate by saying, "The key requirements for principal-care encounters in our survey were an assumption by the

Table 6.7. Percentage of patient encounters in all practice arrangements

Specialty	First	Episodic	Principal	Consultation	Specialized
General practice	10.5	4.9	80.1	2.2	2.4
Family practice	13.1	4.1	77.7	2.7	2.3
Pediatrics	15.5	4.0	72.3	5.3	3.0
Internal medicine	13.2	5.2	61.9	15.3	4.1
Obstetrics/gynecology	13.2	4.0	65.0	6.3	11.4
Cardiology	6.6	5.4	58.2	21.7	8.1
Gastroenterology	9.4	8.3	42.3	34.5	5.6
Pulmonology	10.9	6.4	43.8	31.9	7.0
Allergy	7.5	3.0	32.9	9.0	47.5
Dermatology	23.5	10.7	16.7	6.7	42.4
Endocrinology	12.0	6.3	45.7	25.6	10.4
Infectious disease	11.6	9.8	22.6	54.4	1.7
Rheumatology	9.0	5.6	52.9	16.9	15.5
Otorhinolaryngology	26.3	9.0	22.5	14.7	27.4

Source: Aiken et al., 1979. (Reprinted by permission)

physician of continuing responsibility for the patient and a commitment to meeting the majority of the patient's medical needs
irrespective of their nature." The findings were that principal
care was by no means confined to primary care physicians who are
the most likely candidates for the family doctor role.

As would be expected, high proportions of patient encounters
for general practitioners and family practitioners were classified as principal care (80 percent and 78 percent respectively).
Nor is it surprising that physicians in the specialties of pediatrics, internal medicine, and obstetrics-gynecology should have
high proportions of their patient encounters as principal care
physicians--these specialties are often designated as primary care
(Table 6.7). But physicians in the other specialties were heavily
involved in providing principal care to patients on a longer term
--family doctor--basis. The authors say, ". . . to a surprising
degree, physicians in all specialties are the principal source of
care to a substantial portion of their patients" (Aiken et al.,
1979) and they conclude that conventional labels do not always
correspond with actual practice. The data suggest that "substantial amounts of generalist care can be and are delivered through a
'hidden network' of specialty physicians" (Aiken et al., 1979).
Furthermore, the data are useful in assessing the extent to which
referral patterns indicate informal regionalization. The sequen-
tial progression via a primary care physician as family doctor
through the complex health care system on the basis of professional referral and consultation is not entirely supported by
these data. In this regard, the first data column of Table 6.7 is
quite informative. In the first encounter category "the patient
has not been seen by the physician previously, and the physician's
role is not that of a consultant to another physician" (Aiken et
al., 1979). The data indicate that specialists, not usually
thought of as entry-point physicians, often have patient encounters without referrals from other physicians.

Referrals by family doctors for rural people. A study of physician use in rural Missouri revealed that while most families
reported having a family doctor, the referral pattern departed
substantially from that suggested by the idealized form of doctor-
patient relationship (Hassinger et al., 1970). In the study,
interviews were conducted with the female heads of 951 families
randomly selected in the towns and open country of four rural communities. Eighty-six percent of the families reported having a
family doctor. With few exceptions, family doctors were local
physicians, all of whom were in general practice. The bulk of
physician use was with the person's family doctor, accounting for
70 percent of all doctor visits during the year of the study. Of
the families, 30 percent used only a family doctor during the
year, while 47 percent used the family doctor plus one or more
nonfamily doctors (13 percent used only a nonfamily doctor and 10
percent used no doctor).

It was determined that 564 of the 951 families used a non-

family doctor during the survey year and they reported 1,006 instances of such use. An attempt was made to identify the source
of referral for each of the 1,006 visits. The referral source was
a self-report based on the response to the question, "Who suggested that you see this doctor?" In about 17 percent of the instances in which a nonfamily doctor was used, referral was made by
a family doctor and in about 15 percent by a nonfamily doctor.
Therefore, about one-third of the instances were reported to have
occurred through professional referral. Eleven percent of the referral sources were designated as institutional. These included
referrals from places of employment in cases of accident or illness and, in cases of medical indigency, from public agencies and
local government. Many nonfamily doctors were seen on the advice
of laypersons, especially relatives, friends, and neighbors. Another sizable source of referral was the doctor's reputation,
which may be interpreted as a more generalized form of lay advice.

     In the 449 families that used both a family doctor and one or
more nonfamily doctors during the year, 27 percent reported that
at least one instance of use of a nonfamily doctor was on the
basis of referral from the family doctor.

     Data from this study indicate that the family-doctor rela-
tionship was quite prevalent and the family doctor provided a
large part of the medical care in the community. As a gatekeeper
to the health care system, however, the referral experience of the
family doctor, although not entirely lacking, does not conform
well to expectations. The reasons for this failure are suggested
by the earlier discussion of criteria for the gatekeeper role.

     Professional referral as a mechanism for coordinating health
care delivery applies more precisely to the use of specialists.
In the previous tabulations, physicians to whom patients were referred were not identified as specialists or nonspecialists. Of
the 238 (27 percent) families who used one or more specialists
during the study year, 61 percent reported professional referral
in at least one instance. It should be noted that these are not
necessarily family doctor referrals and that families reporting a
professional referral might, in other instances, have used specialists without such referral. The data, however, do indicate
some professional orderliness in selection and use of specialists
in these rural communities.

     The intention of this chapter was to assess the extent to
which regionalization has occurred in a health care system that is
largely unplanned and unmanaged. In doing this, the elements of
regionalized systems--differentiation, spatial order, and vertical
coordination--were considered. The general conclusion is that the
delivery systems are far from chaotic and do not deserve the term
nonsystem, which is sometimes applied.

     Differentiation in the form of specialization of physicians
and health facilities has unfolded in response to expansion of
knowledge and technology and opportunity to serve an increasingly
demanding clientele.

     There is a certain degree of order in the location of health

services that conforms roughly to marketplace criteria. One does
not expect health services to survive without subsidy in remote
areas where specialized services are found at less frequent spatial intervals than nonspecialized services. Adjustments are
likely to be continuous and incremental.

Coordination of health services depends heavily on providers.
Physicians are the key element in professional referral, which
ideally provides a mechanism to assure appropriate and comprehensive care to patients. The family-doctor relationship institu-
tionalizes this mechanism through mutual obligations and expectations of client and doctor. Although the family-doctor relationship is widely acknowledged, it departs significantly but not
totally from its idealized form.

The unmanaged health care system has many critics. There are
overlaps and gaps in services. Not all segments of society are
served equitably. It is a system subject to wrong emphasis in
promoting a healthy population (i.e., cure versus prevention). It
is a system that cannot contain costs when constraints on use by
individuals are upset by corporate and government financing of
personal health care. Efforts have been made to solve these problems through various forms of planning and organization, which are
examined in the next chapter.

Managed Regionalization
of Health Services

Critics of health care are numerous and vocal. The term "crisis" is frequently invoked to characterize the health care system. The crisis involves such problems as maldistribution of health resources, access to health services, priorities of the health profession, and quality of health services.

A common criticism is lack of equity in obtaining health care. In such a vital area as health services, equity is easily translated into equality. But realities reveal that there are two levels of health care--one geared to the affluent, the other to the poor. The principle of equity also suffers from the maldistribution of services. At base, the allocation of health resources on the basis of marketplace principles is antithetical to equal access to health services.

Furthermore, controls of the market and the profession may not work in the present health care system. A quantum change has occurred in health care organization, with the hospital at its center. The pinnacle in the organization of hospitals is the medical center, which commands large resources, incorporates highly sophisticated technology, provides the most specialized services, engages in teaching and research, and serves a wide-ranging clientele which may be statewide, nationwide, or worldwide. Such enterprises bring together a truly remarkable collection of specialties of high technology. These complex activities require expert management; they also require, as a means of assuring resources, control over their external environment. The process of controlling the external environment of medical centers consists of establishing domain over a set of services and a service area and establishing relationships with other units of the health care system. Short-term and long-term planning are part of this process. On a smaller scale, the same kinds of problems apply to lesser hospitals and other health facilities, and value is placed on the ordering of relationships among units of the health care system. Regionalization is a rational approach to such ordering.

As with unmanaged regionalization, we can consider the elements of managed regionalization by examining (1) the differentia-

tion of services, (2) the spatial ordering of services, and (3)
the means of control. In this task, instead of searching out the
surprising regularities of unmanaged regionalization, we look at
the conscious efforts to plan and implement within the regionalization framework.

DIFFERENTIATION OF MANAGED SERVICES

Physicians
       Until quite recently, public policy in health manpower was
almost nonexistent. The medical profession was accused of placing
severe limitations on the production of physicians, and the development of specialty programs and their selection by students was
without overall planning. Reacting first to the shortage of physicians and then to the disproportionate numbers in certain specialties, the federal government entered manpower policy mainly
through economic incentives. The first thrust was support of new
medical schools, which rose in number from 85 in 1950 to 123 in
1975, and increasing the size of existing medical school classes.
Accompanying these efforts were incentives to train more physicians in the primary care specialties. With the end of the physician shortage, financial incentives to increase the number of physicians have been curtailed, but the stress on training primary
care physicians continues. The Health Resources Administration of
the U.S. Public Health Service has made extensive projections of
health manpower needs to help close the gap between supply of and
need for health manpower.

Physician Extenders
       Of considerable importance is the genre of new health practi-
tioners developed to meet the perceived need for primary care in
situations neglected by physicians. A class referred to as *physician extenders* consists of physician assistants, nurse practitioners, and MEDEX. While not without precedent (for example, the
nurse midwives of the Frontier Nursing Service), the impetus be-
hind the increased importance of physician extenders was a desire
to solve a particular set of problems such as lack of primary care
practitioners and deficiencies of distribution of such practitioners.
       The first program for physician assistants started at Duke
University in 1965. This was at the height of the Vietnam War and
the intention was to utilize the expertise of discharged medical
service corpsmen. Programs for training physician extenders have
risen rapidly. In mid-1975, the Bureau of Health Manpower reported a total of 93 training programs for physician assistants
(these did not include nurse practitioners). Programs ranging
from one to four years were located in 35 states and the District
of Columbia (Bowers, 1977). The American Medical Association
(AMA) house of delegates adopted minimum standards for assistants

to primary care physicians in 1971. Most but not all states have
granted legislative sanctions to physician assistants; however,
regulations regarding supervision are not uniform.

A program that received much attention and has given its name
to a type of physician extender is MEDEX, which started at the
University of Washington in 1969. It provides a 15-month training
program for persons with practical experience in health care, especially discharged medical service corpsmen. Twelve months of
the training is in preceptorship with a physician. While the program is applicable to urban as well as rural areas, most of the
trainees are placed in rural settings with the expectation that
they will remain there as an associate of the physician with whom
they trained.

Nurse practitioners are the most numerous of the physician
extenders, although nurses are not entirely happy with being
classified together with physician assistants. The roots of their
entrance into the practice field extend into public health and
programs in remote areas such as the Frontier Nursing Service of
Kentucky. And even without the emergence of the "practitioner"
designation, the role of nurses has expanded in medical care. In
1971 the Federal Nurse Training Act provided funds to train nurse
practitioners. Nurses have specialized in such practice areas as
pediatrics, nurse-midwives, and family practice. The family nurse
practitioner has received special designation under a federal
training program known as PRIMEX.

As aspirants to professional recognition, physician extenders
have taken certain steps to sharpen identity and establish a niche
in the professional hierarchy. A step toward professionalization
is the accreditation of training programs for physician assistants
by a joint committee of the AMA and the American Academy of Physicians' Assistants; by 1977, 43 programs had been accredited.
Furthermore, the National Board of Medical Examiners in collaboration with the AMA administers an annual examination for the certification of "assistant to the primary care physician." The American Nurses Association (ANA) separately accredits training programs for expanded nursing roles as part of its review and accreditation of nursing schools. The ANA also offers certifying examinations for family nurse practitioners and certification is
available for nurse-midwives and pediatric nurse practitioners.
Nurse practitioners may also take the National Physicians' Assistant Certifying Examination. The professional domains of non-nurse
physician assistants and nurse practitioners have not been fully
worked out and there is some tension between them (Denham and
Pickard, 1979).

A major question that persists is the extent of practice and
the level and conditions of supervision that physician extenders
should have. The term, physician extenders, places the practitioners in a role subordinate to physicians. The range of services that new health practitioners provide has increased over
time.

The care that people seek from new health practitioners is
the care that people seek most of the time--illness prevention such as immunization and health education; management of
simple and common illnesses; monitoring of chronic illnesses
like hypertension and diabetes; complete physicals; prenatal
care of expectant mothers; minor surgery; and emergency
stabilization care for seriously ill or injured people until
they reach an emergency care facility. . . . Simple and common illnesses are not limited to colds and the flu. New
health practitioners are well trained to diagnose and treat a
wide range of children's and adults' diseases, including respiratory infections and urinary tract infections" [Bernstein
et al., 1979].

In studies of practitioners in clinics in which physicians are not
present except for limited times, physician extenders are able to
manage from 70 to 80 percent of the cases that come to the clinic
without further consultation.

The work of the physician extender is illustrated by the case
of a clinic in Nageezi, a remote area in New Mexico. The principal personnel are a full-time physician assistant and a physician
who is present one day a week. The following is from a report
prepared by the physician and the physician assistant.

The designation "trained primary health practitioner" best
describes the role of the Nageezi full-time physician assistant. Much of her day-to-day activity consists of education,
counseling, diagnosis and treatment of patients and families
or clinic administration without physician consultation. Her
independent activities, in fact, comprise more than 90 percent of Nageezi patient encounters. We feel that there is no
need for on-site or remote physician supervision for the vast
majority of patient visits. As quality of these services
cannot be maintained by continuous physician supervision,
periodic chart audit and impromptu physician observation is
substituted. . . . The physician assistant is usually "first
contact" for Nageezi patients and therefore is usually identified as the "family practitioner." The physician, on the
other hand, is present at the clinic only one full day per
week. Much of his time is generally spent seeing more complicated patients by referral and those few patients who re-
quest a doctor. In addition, time is spent teaching the P.A.
[physician assistant] and staff as well as health science
students rotating through the Health System. Finally, the
physician devotes time to chart audit and observation of the
P.A. with the objective of maintaining and improving quality
of care [Kozoll and Poncho, n.d.].

Physician extenders now perform in a wide variety of medical
settings--from the medical center to solo practices in remote
areas. And in most reports they have been found to perform within

their range at a level of competency equal to that of physicians.
There seems to be general acceptance of the new health practitioners by the public if they have the proper practice setting and if
their work is supported by local physicians. The hope that physician extenders would substantially reduce the costs of health
services, however, may not be well founded. A review from the
Congressional Budget Office in 1979 suggests that physician extenders may simply increase the amount of service that people use
and much of the increase in expenditures may be absorbed by physicians who employ the physician extenders. There is some concern
that, as with physicians, physician extenders may create excessive
demand for services, which will result in higher costs for patients.
      In terms of managed regionalization, a consideration of the
creation of types of health practitioners where none existed
before is pertinent. It cannot be said that physician extenders
are a type of practitioner that was demanded by the public or even
by the medical profession. Instead, they were created in response
to problems perceived by planners, educators, and academicians.
Academicians tend to judge the new profession favorably, but the
judgment of the public and the medical profession is still out
(Glenn and Hofmeister, 1976; Fottler et al., 1978).

Primary Health Care Clinics
      Companion to new health practitioners are primary health care
clinics designed to meet the needs of people in remote areas or
other areas where health services are not economically feasible.
These clinics have roots in programs started by the Office of Economic Opportunity (OEO) as part of President Johnson's War on Poverty. Neighborhood health centers were established to provide
primary health care to populations in low income areas of cities
and the country. They tended to be areas of considerable size and
represented substantial efforts to meet the needs of the most
needy people. The centers were conscious of the health implications of the poverty environment and often supported community
programs in sanitation, nutrition, and employment. One of the
purposes of the centers was to train and employ persons indigenous
to the area. The centers also stressed lay participation in the
policy decisions.
      Although usually associated with urban areas, neighborhood
health centers were established in rural areas--especially in the
rural South. The first of the rural centers was the Tufts-Delta
Health Center at Mound Bayou, Bolivar County, Mississippi. Tufts
University School of Medicine, Boston, undertook the development
of a program to provide comprehensive primary health services.
The location was one of the most depressed in the nation, and
truly shocking statistics were reported to support the need for
the program. When the organizational effort began, the average
family income was less than $1,000 per year and the infant mor-
tality rate was more than twice that of the nation (Geiger, 1969).
A survey found serious health problems among the almost wholly

black population, including malnutrition and conditions that modern medicine has long been able to conquer. Dramatic attention was drawn to the nutritional problem after the center was established by billing OEO for food in the form of prescriptions as a specific remedy for hunger. In November 1967, after almost three years of planning, the center was opened in a remodeled church parsonage. Late in 1968, a new facility was opened. It consisted of a 24,000 square foot building where office space was provided for three family care groups, each consisting of an internist, a pediatrician, a general practitioner, community health nurses, nurses' aides, and sanitarians. Additional space was available for an obstetrician-gynecologist, a surgeon, and a psychologist who served all three groups. Also, there was an emergency room and other facilities including a delivery room, X-ray facilities, record room, lab, and pharmacy.

A feature of the Tufts-Delta Center was the involvement of local people in the program. This was done in two ways. The center employed many local people on its staff and had a program for training them as nurses' aides and home health aides. Also, local health associations were organized in the several neighborhoods of the area, which in turn had representation on an areawide health planning council. The council was involved in setting priorities and in planning the health center program.

The health center became involved with the community in other ways. Observing that many people in the area were struggling to get minimum food, clothing, and shelter, and since these things are essential in promoting health, a cooperative farm and cooperative grocery and clothing outlets were started. Furthermore, the areawide health council became involved in a water sanitation project, a housing program, and a project for patient transportation (Hatch and Earp, 1976).

Tufts University's relationship with the center ended in 1972. Under OEO mandate, merger plans between the center and Mound Bayou Hospital were initiated. With the merger, the center serves as an outpatient facility. In a sense the merger was a victory for the political and medical elite of Mound Bayou, which had resented the outside influence of an eastern medical school and the involvement of the poor in somewhat unusual solutions to social problems.

The federal program of support for primary health centers continued with the Community Health Centers program, which is a combination of three earlier programs (Neighborhood Health Centers, Family Health Centers, and Community Health Network). Emphasis was shifted to support smaller and more limited programs, but 158 of the earlier larger projects (including Mound Bayou) were still supported under this program in 1978 and consumed about 80 percent of the funds available.

Smaller primary care centers in rural areas are typically staffed by physician extenders, with off-site consultation by physicians. Such clinics have had to carve a niche for themselves in the health delivery system in terms of acceptance by the public,

the health profession, and the legal system. A major step in the
legitimation of the centers was the passage in 1977 of the Rural
Health Clinic Services Act (PL 95-210), which specified that services of midlevel health practitioners without on-site supervision
of a physician were eligible for reimbursement from Medicare and
Medicaid. The legislation also specified requirements for certification of primary clinics. Further evidence of efforts to establish a place in the health delivery system for rural primary
care clinics is the organization of the National Rural Primary
Care Association. The association seeks to promote and serve as a
clearinghouse for rural clinics. Its most important activity is
to bring organized pressure on the federal government for support.
    North Carolina has pioneered in the development of new health
practitioner primary health clinics. Legislation created the
Office of Rural Health Services in 1973 and mandated the development of five primary care clinics the first year and five more the
second. By 1977, 17 community-sponsored new health practitioner
clinics had been built. The new health practitioner clinic is
seen as part of the larger system. "Such a practice functions as
an extension of the larger health care system in the surrounding
commercial or medical community. It provides a doorway for people
to obtain appropriate health care conveniently at the local level
and assures access to more complex care when needed" (Bernstein et
al., 1979).
    The regionalization features of this model can be seen in the
following statement.

    Of key importance to the health center's potential for suc-
    cess is the new health practitioner's access to a referral
    network in the area. Independently or through the back-up
    physician, the new health practitioner must be able to refer
    patients to appropriate specialists for more complex diagno-
    sis and treatment. In many cases, appointments with special-
    ists are arranged for the patient by the new practitioners,
    especially if the need is urgent. Community residents are
    thus assured of access to whatever level of care they may
    need [Bernstein et al., 1979].

    Another model of rural primary practice that has received
attention is the Rural Practice Project directed by Donald Madison. It is a demonstration project in which the Robert Wood Johnson Foundation provides initial planning and start-up funds to
develop rural practice clinics. The project looks for innovation
in health delivery and its goal is to establish a self-sustaining
practice that (1) has two or more physicians working as a team
with non-physician health practitioners and (2) exhibits sound and
advanced management techniques. Many of the ideas that went into
the model were derived from the experience of a successful rural
clinic in eastern Kentucky. Started by a physician-administrator
team, the clinic has expanded its staff to four physicians, six
nurse practitioners, a pharmacist, and an X-ray technician. The

service area has been extended by building a clinic at a second
site (Henig, 1976).

An illustration of the model is a clinic organized to serve
about 12,000 residents of four small towns, an Indian reservation,
and the open country of north central Minnesota. The initiative
for the project was taken by a young physician, native to Minnesota, who gained the support of the community and assembled a
staff. The clinic is a nonprofit corporation, which owns and op-
erates the practice. An advisory board of local citizens has substantial policy input to the clinic. The staff is projected to
consist of three physicians, a nurse practitioner, a physician
assistant, a pharmacist, a mental health worker, and a social
worker. All of the staff, including the physicians, are salaried.
Reliance on nonphysician staff members is a hallmark of the Rural
Health Project. The initial facility is a converted garage in one
of the small towns. There are plans for a second clinic at another place. Arrangements have been made to use the facilities of a
local 80-bed hospital and services on referral of a multispecialty
group practice in suburban Minneapolis (Rural Practice Project,
1976).

A review of rural projects for the delivery of primary health
services, of which there are some 1,500, revealed five practice
models (Sheps and Bachar, 1981).

- *Community Health Centers*--Comprehensive programs of a relatively large scale together with substantial community involvement
and control. The range of services is broad and includes non-
clinical support services. Examples are neighborhood health centers and family health centers such as Mound Bayou.
- *Organized Group Practices*--These programs place emphasis on
leadership, sophisticated administration, and staff development.
The basic structure calls for at least two full-time primary care
providers sharing facilities, income, and support staff. The
Rural Practice Model of the Robert Wood Foundation is illustrative
of this type.
- *Freestanding Primary Care Center*--These programs result
from community initiative and continued involvement with or without government or foundation support. They usually start with one
physician or new health practitioner. These units tend to be
smaller and provide less extensive services than community health
centers. Examples are numerous and widely spread across the
nation.
- *Traditional Solo Practices*--The emphasis is on placement of
medical and allied manpower in areas of need. Less attention is
given to health programs, administration, linkages with other
health units, and technical assistance. The primary example is
the National Health Service Corps.
- *Institutional Extended Program Model*--Services for rural
populations developed by existing institutions such as hospitals,
health departments, and group practices. Rural satellites from
medical centers or established group practices are examples.

The models indicate that serious attention is being given to
developing health service organizations appropriate for rural situations. The seriousness of the attempt to provide appropriate
primary health services and to join them in a systematic manner to
the larger health care system is also apparent in the federal government's Rural Health Initiative (RHI) program. It seeks to integrate a number of programs as they apply to rural areas, including community health centers, the Migrant Health Program, the
Appalachian Health Program, and the National Health Service Corps.
Program guidance material of RHI indicates a regionalization
approach. While efforts of RHI are devoted almost exclusively to
providing primary care to underserved rural areas, emphasis is
placed on the concept of a larger integrated system. One of the
goals reads:

> To identify and make maximum use of existing health care re-
> sources, by using new approaches and concepts directed at
> combining, coordinating, and strengthening health service
> delivery resources and activities through establishment of
> linkages between primary, secondary, and tertiary care
> [USDHEW, 1978b].

SPATIAL ORDERING OF MANAGED SERVICES

Health Manpower
The official line in health manpower policy is that the physician shortage has ended and a glut of physicians is a distinct
possibility. Similarly, hospital beds are in ample supply and
their excess is blamed as a factor in the high costs of health
services. However, the distribution of health resources continues
to be a problem, but even this is not a unitary problem. Physi-
cian/population ratios continue to be skewed dramatically toward
metropolitan areas. The hospital situation, however, is different. Rural areas, thanks to Hill-Burton, have reached rough parity with urban areas in hospital beds/population ratios. The
problem in this case is that small rural hospitals have a difficult time maintaining adequate bed censuses, many of which are below 50 percent. In a sense, the marketplace has defeated the
planners.
William Rushing (1975) views maldistribution of physicians as
a problem of organization. He is not optimistic that increasing
the supply of physicians will affect maldistribution, since afflu-
ent-urbanized areas can absorb more physicians and a larger number of physicians may *create* greater demand. He does see promise
for a regionalized system in attracting, and retaining, manpower
to a rural area. "It is suggested that intercommunity medical
networks be established around a community that, because of its
social and economic resources, and in combination with the population of surrounding communities, could support a viable medical
community. . . . Referral systems would be developed, or systema-

tized where they now exist, between physicians in the central community and physicians in outlying communities."

Rosemary Stevens is not optimistic either about attempts to
rationalize the distribution of health manpower. A major problem,
as she sees it, is that health facilities are often equated with
health services. Thus in the minds of many planners and decision
makers, health services have become a world of buildings. "It is
only a step from here to the notion, implicit in all health planning legislation to this date, that the regulation of buildings
will lead to the regulation of the entire health service industry"
(Stevens, 1977).

If this were in fact true, it would be relatively easy to
control the distribution of health personnel.

> The employer would decide how many personnel were required in
> each category to serve a particular population, and would
> hire, fire and remunerate accordingly. The allocation of
> funding to a regional health consortium, channeled through
> its institutions, would thus have a direct impact on the dis-
> tribution of health manpower in that area, and in relation to
> other areas. For example, a regional health agency might
> decide to employ more nurse practitioners as a partial sub-
> stitute for physicians in primary care. Since, under this
> scheme, the organization would have an effective monopoly of
> the job market in medical care, this decision would expand
> the demand for nurse practitioners in the area and reduce the
> demand for primary physicians. In areas in which the demand
> for primary physicians was met, there would be no job open-
> ings; physicians would have to practice somewhere else. In
> aggregate, there would thus be a shifting of personnel within
> and across regions according to the supply of available jobs
> [Stevens, 1977].

Stevens notes that this neat and tidy picture bears little
relation to the way in which health manpower is actually distributed. To depend on health facilities to provide a rational distribution of personnel for health services is a distorted view of
the power of the industry.

> While hospitals are the major employers of health employees,
> they are by no means the only employer. Health workers are
> employed in the country's 20,000 nursing homes, in health
> maintenance organizations, in home health agencies, in the
> Veterans Administration, in Indian Health Services, and in
> many other services, programs, and institutions. Many health
> workers are self-employed: pharmacists, dentists, optome-
> trists, and physicians. The combined result is not an indus-
> trial employment situation that could be rationalized into
> national, regional, and local units through the structure of
> employment per se. It is rather a hodgepodge of profession-

als, technicians, clerical workers, and others, clustered in
different settings. The physician in his or her private
office, the pharmacist in the drugstore, the nurse in a visiting nurse association, the laboratory technologist working
for a private laboratory service, the dentist and dental
hygienist, the podiatrist, the optometrist, and others in
their offices are all essential elements in the provision of
comprehensive health services, and all are elements that cannot be effectively regulated through health care buildings
and facilities [Stevens, 1977].

Stevens suggests some methods through which health manpower
might be allocated to achieve distributions compatible with regionalization and which she says are technically possible but not
politically feasible.

• Hospitals could be required to offer admitting and other
staff privileges to only those physicians whose presence could be
justified by community "need" as defined by each local Health Systems Agency (HSA). Since most physicians rely on hospital affiliation, such restrictions could be potent. If a physician seeking
to practice orthopedics in a particular area were denied a hospital staff position, he or she would be bereft of the means to pursue a career. The alternatives would be to change specialty or go
elsewhere. Doctors would be discouraged from entering practice in
specialties and/or locations well supplied with physicians. Regionalized medical services would be achieved relatively pain-
lessly with the responsibility for planning clearly assigned to
HSAs.
• The power to license physicians, dentists, pharmacists,
optometrists, and others might be made contingent on practice in
specific agencies or locations. National licensure arrangements
might also be developed with specific manpower goals in view. In
well-served areas the available licensing "slots" would be used up
and practitioners would be deflected to work elsewhere.
• Stevens then moves to an even more extreme suggestion. She
says, "Once the Federal Government has distorted the market system
by intervening in the field in as massive a way as it has done,
the logical answer to rational distribution might be complete Federal control of professional locations. Whatever the form of regulation, the most effective way of insuring that health manpower
is relatively evenly and efficiently spread across the population
would be for government or its agents to monopolize health care
jobs. In a national health service, jobs would be made available
only where justified by regional economic priorities and/or planning criteria" (Stevens, 1977).
• Such controls of manpower distribution clearly are not currently feasible. Stevens mentions a number of efforts that were
designed at least in part to distribute health personnel in a rational and equitable manner. Among these are Health Maintenance

Organizations (HMOs), Professional Standards Review Organizations
(PSROs), HSAs, Area Health Education Centers (AHECs), and the National Health Service Corps. These "solutions," however, she
characterizes as "puny and partial."

As a case in point, considerable hope has been attached to
HMOs as means of ordering the distribution of health services.

The HMO is a self-contained, locally run health service
system. Offering defined health services on a prepaid
basis to an enrolled service group, it must balance the
costs of its benefits to subscribers against the costs of
personnel and other expenditures. There is a built-in
planning system in each HMO, which does not exist in other
forms of private practice, the incentive to develop staffing patterns to meet limited and specific services. That
was part of the appeal of HMOs when the notion surfaced in
1970. If the HMO became the dominant pattern of medical
care for all persons in the United States (a hope that was
then optimistically expressed), decisions about health care
costs and resources would be decentralized to the local
level. . . . Manpower decisions would be taken by each organization, and there would be less call for other regional
systems of manpower surveillance and/or regulation. If the
great majority of the population were served by self-contained health service systems, there would be no room for
physicians or other independent practitioners above the
service requirements of each system. Inevitably, then,
HMOs would have some effect on the redistribution of health
manpower from area to area and region to region. Blanket-
ed together over the Nation, HMOs could form an interlocking network of independent health care systems [Stevens,
1977].

Stevens notes, "The heady prospects of 1970, however, have
had little impact on the real world." She attributes this to the
stringency of federal regulations, which has made it difficult to
compete with traditional health insurance plans. And she finds
that the HMO has moved conceptually from a potential for health
care reorganization on a massive scale to an alternative system of
delivery in certain areas. The regional manpower implications of
HMOs are, at best, underdeveloped, for even in areas with HMOs
there is extensive room for independent practitioners (Stevens,
1977).

Renewed activity in HMOs has indeed occurred, as Stevens has
suggested it might, with relaxation of federal requirements and
increasing concern of governments and employers for rising costs.
Special dispensations from HSA regulations have been given to HMOs
that would serve rural populations. In the Twin Cities of Minnesota, HMOs have made a significant impact, with reports that about
75 percent of the physicians and most of the hospitals are participants. But a modification has occurred in the concepts that
would appear to substantially alter the effect on distribution of

personnel. Many of the physicians participating in HMOs also retain fee-for-service practices. This diminishes the impact of
HMOs on physician location and commitment of physicians to the HMO
principles.

Identifying medically underserved areas and health manpower shortage areas. The most direct effort of the federal government to
change the distribution of health personnel, and one which has
special relevance for rural areas, is identifying areas with deficiencies in health services and directing personnel and programs
to them. Two principal designations are made--Medically Underserved Areas (MUAs) and Health Manpower Shortage Areas (HMSAs).
Community health centers require location in MUAs for federal
funding and preference is given to support of HMOs so located.
National Health Service Corps placements are in HMSAs, and a requirement for Medicare and Medicaid reimbursement to rural health
clinics with no physician present is location in a MUA or HMSA.
      MUAs are designated on the basis of an Index of Medical Un-
derservice (IMU), which was developed by researchers at the University of Wisconsin. The IMU consists of four variables: ratio
of primary care physicians to population, infant mortality rate,
percent of population below the poverty level, and percent of the
population 65 years and over.
      HMSAs were originally based on selected practitioner/popula-
tion ratios for areas (usually counties). Additional criteria
were specified later pertaining to delineating rational service
areas, varying care needs of populations, and consideration of
manpower available in contiguous areas.
      HMSAs are identified for seven manpower types, which include
primary medical care manpower (including primary care physicians,
nurse practitioners, and physician assistants); dental manpower;
pharmacy manpower; and veterinary manpower (Lee, 1979). Most of
the HMSAs are in nonmetropolitan areas as shown in Table 7.1. In
urban areas, almost all the HMSAs involve access problems rather
than an absence of primary care physicians. Most of these access
problems are economic, often aggravated by racial, cultural, or
language differences (Lee, 1979).

The National Health Service Corps. The National Health Service
Corps (NHSC) has become a key program in the managed distribution
of health services. The program, initiated by legislation in
1971, involves awarding scholarships, recruiting, and placing
health professionals. Scholarships are awarded to professional
health students (physicians, nurses, nurse practitioners, physician assistants, dentists, and allied health practitioners), with
an obligation to practice one year for each scholarship year in a
health manpower shortage area. Most, but not all, the recruits
come from scholarship recipients. The NHSC provides salaried
health professionals as well as administrative and management assistance to communities. The community agrees to manage the NHSC

Table 7.1. Health manpower shortage area designations, January 10–September 30, 1978

Type of designation Geographic area	Primary medical care	Dentistry	Psychiatry*	Optometry	Pharmacy	Podiatry	Veterinary medicine Companion animal	Large animal
Inner urban	101	29	1	14+	3+	334+	12+	34+
Other metropolitan	202	8	...	201	138	747	96	604
Nonmetropolitan	858	455	61	...	...	...	...	...
Population group	22	6	...	...	...	...	...	...
Facility	5	1	...	...	...	...	...	...
Total	1,188	499	62	215	141	1,081	108	638

Source: Lee, 1979.

*For psychiatric manpower shortage areas, this category is defined as containing some metropolitan areas.

+Metropolitan area.

practice; provide an office, supplies, and staff support; and is
responsible for purchasing, billing, and collecting fees (Kane et
al., 1979). Most of the assignments of NHSC personnel are to rural areas for two-year periods, which may be renewed. It is hoped
that recruits will remain in the area after their service obligations have been fulfilled, although the early record of the corps
is not encouraging on this score.

     The NHSC proved to be popular with Congress and in 1976 the
size of the corps and the scholarship program were increased substantially. In the fiscal year 1979-1980, 5,370 medical and osteopathic students were receiving scholarship support (9 percent of
the nation's medical students) and another 3,000 were deferred
from service pending completion of residency training. In 1979
the corps had about 1,000 physicians in community practices (Mullan, 1980). Provisions in the 1976 legislation also made it much
more difficult for scholarship students to default on their service obligations--the pay back penalty is triple the amount of
scholarship support. Donald Madison and Budd Shenkin (1980) say,
"This formerly peripheral program has now become the centerpiece
of a national strategy to serve the underserved."

Facilities
     Spatial plans appear to be more uniform and precise for re-
gionalization of health facilities than for health personnel.
Characteristically, different levels of facilities are identified
and related spatially to each other in a planetary manner. It
makes little difference if the plans develop from the national
level downward or from the local level upward; the spatial ordering is similar. Entry points (primary health centers) are related to specific hospitals providing secondary level services, which
in turn are related to specific medical centers of tertiary level
services. The pattern of four levels (an extra hospital level is
identified) the U.S. Public Health Service developed prior to the
Hill-Burton legislation was shown in Chapter Four (Fig. 4.1).
Furthermore, diagrams of the Russian (Shannon and Dever, 1974) and
Swedish (Werko, 1971) spatial organizations are similar, as is the
Cuban system drawn from the following description by Milton
Roemer (1976b):

     The keystone of the system is the local polyclinic, serving
     about 25,000 to 30,000 people in what is called a health
     service area. It serves these people for primary care, medi-
     cal and dental care, preventive services, and emergencies.
     There are about three hundred of these polyclinics throughout
     the island, staffed by salaried teams of doctors and allied
     health workers, to serve 9 million people.
         Some seven or eight service areas are linked to make up
     a health region, which contains typically between 200,000 and
     250,000 people. There are about forty of these health re-
     gions throughout Cuba, each headed by a public health physi-
     cian. The polyclinics are headed by a qualified physician

who has had some public health training. Each health region
is provided also with a regional or district hospital, where
the services of specialists are available for both outpatient
and inpatient care.

Five or six health regions comprise what they speak of
as a health province, of which there are eight in Cuba. Politically, Cuba has six governmental provinces, but two of
them, Havana and Oriente, are divided into two parts. At the
provincial level is the most highly developed hospital, with
the most highly trained specialists for tertiary care, as
well as services for secondary care for the adjacent population.

If the patterns of spatial organization of health services
suggested by regionalization plans are compared with the idealized
pattern of service centers that result from marketing principles
as developed by Christaller, one might conclude that the spatial
organization of health planners simply formalized the pattern of
location on the basis of marketing principles. The relationship
among service units of managed and unmanaged regionalization is
different, however. In marketplace relationships, the locations
of higher level service divide the areas of lower level service.
Thus the area of each lower level is divided among three higher
level centers (see Fig. 6.1). A different principle applies to
the location of service units in the managed regionalized models
that have just been discussed. The lower level units are connected with higher level units, and the highest level unit has an exclusive area that incorporates the entire service areas of all
service units within its orbit (see Fig. 4.1). Although Christaller was primarily concerned with location on the basis of marketing principles, he accounted for this pattern on the basis of
what he called the administrative principle. In it, lower level
centers are oriented to one and only one higher level center; thus
it abandons the marketing principle of interlocking competition
among three higher level centers. The image, then, is a planetary
model, with the sun, planets, and moons representing three or more
levels of health services.

CONTROL IN MANAGED REGIONALIZATION

Attention is now turned to the organizational aspects--the
control--of this type of regionalization. Regionalization represents a major tool of managers and planners as they seek to bring
order in the delivery of health services. The organizational
forms are quite varied, ranging from the voluntary associations of
peers as found in regional hospital councils to hierarchical controls that change an interorganizational field into a corporate
unit. The processes of control in interorganizational fields were
examined in Chapter Five. The managed types of control were identified as mediated fields, empires, and corporate guided fields.
In the following discussion an attempt is made to examine actual

situations within that conceptual framework. Needless to say,
there is not a perfect fit between typology and concrete cases.

Coordination by Peers--Mediated Fields
     Coordination by peers is a relatively weak mechanism of con-
trol. According to Basil Mott (1971), peer group coordination
lacks authority over members, and the control that coordinating
councils have over member agencies is limited largely to the benefits that members derive from voluntarily cooperating with each
other.

Hospital councils. Councils of hospitals and hospital consortia
are prime examples of mediating mechanisms, as are more broadly
based health and welfare councils. Their activities frequently
center on surveys and planning as well as sharing services and ex-
changing information. David Pearson (1976) points out that professional health practitioners often support this approach. Thus
the American Hospital Association's Commission on Financing Hospital Care, while advocating regionalization, placed emphasis on
voluntary cooperation rather than on mandatory approaches and indicated that "formalization of cooperative actions should result
from a process of natural growth rather than from imposition of
formal organization" (Pearson, 1976). The model cited by the commission was the Rochester Regional Hospital Council, which had
"promoted hospital cooperation in such areas as joint purchasing,
training of interns and nurses, recruitment of personnel, effective reimbursement from public agencies, joint surveys of community needs, and limitation of certain specialized services to specific hospitals" (Pearson, 1976).
     In commenting on consortia among rural hospitals, Richard
Johnson (1978), president of Tribrook management consultants,
says,

     The consortium approach probably has the greatest appeal and
     the weakest organizational structure. In most cases, the ex-
     pectations of the hospitals that have entered consortiums
     never have been fulfilled. In consortiums, the hospitals not
     only are the consumers of the service but are represented on
     the governing boards as well. This organization puts the
     hospitals' representatives in an untenable position, because
     they often are forced to respond to the interests of each
     member rather than the interests of the group as a whole.
     Voluntary consortiums, from which a member can withdraw at
     any time, tend to work only as long as they never have to say
     "no" to any members. Having no means of mandating group de-
     cisions, they usually fall apart or become only "paper" or-
     ganizations.

     Hospital councils may evolve from weak coordinating groups to
agencies that have responsibilities and legal authority for planning. For example, the Rochester Regional Hospital Council became

the state's planning agency for the Rochester area, and the Health and Hospital Planning Council of Southern New York became, for a time, the Comprehensive Health Planning "b" agency for metropolitan New York under federal legislation.

Regionalization of rural health units in Michigan. Weak intervention to advance regionalization among rural health units in Michigan was the subject of an intensive analysis by Walter McNerney and Donald Riedel (1962). The setting was three small primary health care centers in Michigan with service area populations of from 3,800 to 10,000. Emphasis was placed on ambulatory services, but a limited number of hospital beds (10, 18, and 19) were insisted on by community residents. As a condition of financial support, the W. K. Kellogg Foundation required that the three small health facilities (health centers) formally agree to coordinate their activities with two larger hospitals within a framework of regionalization. The signed agreements provided for cooperative arrangements between the medical staffs of the health centers and the hospitals and between the administrative and technical staffs of the health centers and the hospitals and provided for cooperative purchasing of supplies.

The effort and resources the Kellogg Foundation expended to develop the three rural health centers within a framework of regionalization was in a sense a practical application of the recommendations of the Michigan Health Survey of 1946 in which the Foundation participated financially. The report states that health and medical service centers and small community hospitals should be affiliated with the larger hospitals of the region. The report also emphasized the voluntary nature of regional arrangements (McNerney and Riedel, 1962).

Two of the small health centers (18 and 19 beds) were linked in an agreement with a 160-bed hospital 40 miles away; the other small health center (10 beds) was linked with a 226-bed hospital 25 miles away. One of the centers, similar to those in the other communities, consisted of 19 inpatient beds, four doctors' suites, a laboratory and X-ray suite, an emergency room, a laundry and kitchen, an obstetrical suite, and a public lobby (McNerney and Riedel, 1962). In each case, the W. K. Kellogg Foundation contributed a substantial amount of the construction cost and provided payment to cover the cost of all medical, technical, and administrative consultation and assistance rendered as a result of the affiliation for a period of three years.

After four or five years the authors concluded that regionalization had failed. The local health centers remained independent of each other and of the hospitals. The authors report that the most effective degree of affiliation took place at the administrative level. "The administrators of the regional hospitals attended health center board and executive committee meetings faithfully at no small personal sacrifice. At these meetings, they provided the centers with a great deal of useful advice. Too often, however, the health center board members, after indicating receptivity at the board meeting, would not follow through and implement the advice" (McNerney and Riedel, 1962). Although the affiliation agreement had anticipated interchange of personnel between the local centers and the regional hospitals, such visits were extremely rare. The fault was in both directions: the local health center personnel seldom visited the regional centers, and regional center personnel did not visit the health centers. The physicians in two of the centers had only courtesy staff privileges at the regional hospital with which they were affiliated. The regional hospital had a tightly organized staff and it was difficult for outsiders to break in. In fact, the association of one of the local health centers was greater with a hospital not in the regionalized health services framework. Most patient referrals were to that hospital, and doctors associated with that hospital provided coverage for the local physician. Physicians in the third local health center had associate staff privileges at their affiliated regional hospital, and in general the relationships were closer.

In purchasing, another traditional area of activities, the regionalization framework did not advance joint efforts. After several very limited attempts, joint purchasing was abandoned. The authors say, "In essence regionalization, with its signed agreements, remained, on the whole, a paper achievement" (McNerney and Riedel, 1962).

The failure seemed to rest with the local units more than with the larger regional hospitals. Although apparently there was no overwhelming sentiment by the staffs of the regional hospitals for the program, the administrators were sympathetic to the idea and devoted some time and resources to the effort. The local centers, on the other hand, were concerned with developing units with more complete services. For example, the Kellogg Foundation planners were desirous of having an exclusively outpatient facility at one of the sites; however, the local board used the foundation's financial support to expand the facility to include inpatient beds. This kind of local manipulation led the authors to conclude that "there was strong evidence that regionalization was accepted as a stepping stone to autonomy instead of away from it" (McNerney and Riedel, 1962).

Rural health councils. In rural areas during the 1950s a movement developed to promote local (often county) health councils as counterparts to urban health and welfare councils. The effort was to bring health and lay leaders together to examine health problems and develop and implement short-range and long-range plans. Although regionalization was not the focus of most health councils' activities, the efforts were multilevel in that local, state, and national health council organizations existed and local health councils were seen as mechanisms for tapping resources beyond the community's boundaries. Bruce Morgan and Robert McKim (1976) assess the effort as a failure. Rural health councils, they point out, were usually organized by outsiders—a state health council, a university, or more likely a state health department seeking lo-

cal support for its programs. Typically a "mass meeting" (which
was poorly attended) was called to discuss the health problems of
the community and the inability of existing organizations to meet
the needs. This was commonly followed by some type of survey that
had as an objective the involvement of key community people in
council activities as well as documentation of local health care
delivery system inadequacies. The county health council, made up
of representatives from health and health-interested groups, was
to be a coordinating agency to help resolve the inadequacies identified.

Short-range programs (for example, immunization programs,
health screening clinics, health information programs) and long-
range programs (comprehensive health planning, development of a
county health system, attracting and retaining health manpower)
were to be developed by the council. Morgan and McKim (1976) comment that the long-term program goals were rarely achieved. In
many cases the attention of the rural councils was on survival,
and even in that they were not successful. In some places there
undoubtedly are successful organizations of this type, but the
hope of the health council movement as a principal means of coordinating rural health services is dead. It was never fully em-
braced by health professionals and health organizations (such as
the cancer society or heart association) of the counties. In many
instances health councils were used by state health departments or
other outside agencies in a manipulative way to implement a program at the local level. In Missouri, for example, local health
councils were often formed by the state health department to support tax referenda to establish local health departments.

Councils tended to wax and wane on the basis of success of
individual projects rather than on their ability to achieve long-
range goals. With completion of a project (such as support of a
referendum) it became difficult to maintain public interest. And
as the organization started to decline, the interest of local
leaders waned. All the efforts were directed toward keeping the
organization alive--a strategy that was doomed to failure. "In
some counties, county health councils languished for a year or
more without having any meetings before anyone even noticed!"
(Morgan and McKim, 1976).

Rural Health Centers--Empires in the Making

A case of failure. The account of the failed attempt at regionalization of three local health centers in Michigan occurred in the
1950s. One might suppose that over time the idea would be more
compelling and the lessons learned would assure success. However,
some of the same underlying causes for failure were shown in a recent account from a small Kentucky community where a primary care
center was established in association with a university medical
center (Cowen et al., 1976).

A small community in Kentucky, a county seat of about 1,900
population serving a total population of about 8,000, was ap-

proaching a crisis with the imminent loss of two elderly physicians. Their practices were based at a small hospital of 30 beds.
The University of Kentucky, Department of Community Medicine, developed a program designed to meet the needs of the community. It
consisted of a primary health care center (staffed initially from
the Department of Community Medicine) that emphasized physician
workups, health education, use of physician extenders, and ambulatory care. The center was housed in the hospital, sharing its
X-ray and laboratory facilities. Success was achieved in recruiting two young physicians who were expected to come to the center
shortly. The primary care center was soon seeing a large number
of patients.

However, one of the outcomes of the new program, with its
emphasis on outpatient services, was that hospital utilization
dropped significantly below preprimary care center levels. This
was a serious problem. With the reduced census, the community
needed to borrow heavily to keep the hospital open. Then, in a
turn of events, the physicians recruited by the center decided to
enter private practice in the community on a fee-for-service basis. The health center administrator, who was shared with the
hospital, resigned from his center position and the primary care
center was "obliged" to leave the hospital facility. The center
volume declined precipitously as patients turned to the young physicians, whose practice followed the old pattern of brief office
visits and frequent hospitalization.

The authors of the article viewed the problem as a discrepancy in outlook between the university planners and the community.

> The community representatives, although they probably did not
> fully understand it, accepted and participated in early de-
> velopments of the program. It represented "action" and a po-
> tential hope for some sort of resolution of their immediate,
> rather pressing health care problems. However, when the lo-
> cal community was presented with what it felt the community
> needed--two young physicians--the community representatives
> moved rapidly and effectively. They recruited these physi-
> cians to office fee-for-service medicine and filled their
> hospital with patients [Cowen et al., 1976].

The place of the hospital in the community was a key to the
failure of the primary care center. The hospital was an important
source of outside money in this small rural county and the primary
care center diverted resources from it. The traditional pattern
of delivery is

> well designed to harvest federal and state health dollars
> while at the same time limiting and protecting local and pri-
> vate expenditures. Medicaid and Medicare pay most office
> visits at the same rate, regardless of duration, thorough-
> ness, or necessity; they pay inadequately for time-consuming,
> diagnostic evaluations. Many brief visits with simple labo-

ratory and therapeutic procedures were the rule. Because
complete office workups are not adequately covered and,
therefore, are a direct cost to the patients, and because
poor patients cannot pay physicians easily, these types of
services are minimized. Because Medicaid and Medicare pay
the doctor, the pharmacy, and the hospital when the patient
is hospitalized, the number and duration of hospitalization
tended to be maximized [Cowen et al., 1976].

Cases of success. Some of the success stories in rural health
care systems result from the development of strong local units,
which on the one side are able to relate from a position of
strength to medical centers providing tertiary services and on the
other side are able to monopolize the health care of a given area,
which is often extended through satellite facilities. These medical care organizations exhibit some of the characteristics of
health empires.
   The Hunterdon Medical Center--This example of such a facility
is described in detail in the next chapter.[1] It is a system built
around a community health center that delivers a wide range of
services including some but not all tertiary level services. It
also has strong community programs of social service and rehabilitation. Hunterdon has maintained formal relationships with university health centers since its beginning and has extended its
reach into the community and expanded its catchment area through
satellite primary care facilities. In the process it has effectively excluded other practitioners and facilities from its area.
The form is repeated in other well-known hospital/health centers
that have grown up in nonmetropolitan areas. Among them are the
Marshfield Clinic in Marshfield, Wisconsin (population 17,000),
and the Geisinger Medical Center in Danville, Pennsylvania (population 6,000).
   The Marshfield Clinic--The Marshfield Clinic is the dominant
health facility in north central Wisconsin. Established in 1916,
it is now a 175-physician multispecialty group. Clinic physicians
staff St. Joseph's Hospital, a 520-bed general acute hospital
owned and operated by the Sisters of the Sorrowful Mother. A
third unit of the center is the Marshfield Medical Foundation,
which is devoted to research. The clinic is the sixth largest
private multispecialty group practice in the United States. Physicians represent almost all specialties and are full-time salaried employees of the clinic. The clinic qualifies as an HMO
through sponsorship of a prepaid health plan (the Greater Marshfield Community Health Plan) in conjunction with St. Joseph's Hospital and Wisconsin Blue Cross and Surgical Care-Blue Shield. The
prepaid plan has some 54,000 enrollees (over half of those eligible) within a 40-mile radius of Marshfield. The clinic derives

---

   1. The case study of Hunterdon Medical Center is placed in a
separate section in order not to interrupt the narrative line.

about 23 percent of its gross revenue from the Health Plan. The
remainder of the practice is fee-for-service.
    The clinic has expanded its service area through six satel-
lite clinics--two with associated local hospitals--located from 10
to 100 miles from Marshfield. An information bulletin from the
Marshfield Clinic says, "For the physician who wants a primary
care practice in a small town, yet feels the need for major group
affiliation and backup, the outreach centers may provide the best
of both worlds" (Marshfield Clinic, n.d.). The clinic extends its
influence through a number of services to area hospitals and physicians. These include:

    ● EKG--Automated systems utilizing telecommunication (via
data phone), telecopiers, and a computer are provided to 46 hospitals and clinics in Wisconsin, Minnesota, Michigan, and Iowa.
    ● Remote Cardiac Monitoring--Remote, continuous cardiac moni-
toring lets patients in other hospitals benefit from cardiac ex-
perts and equipment in Marshfield.
    ● Clinical Laboratory--Clinical laboratory specimens are cur-
rently received from over 80 medical institutions through shared
services.
    ● Consultation--Psychiatry, psychology, psychiatric social
services, and neurology consultation services are being utilized
by several facilities in north central Wisconsin.
    ● Nuclear Medicine--Scanning and laboratory operation consul-
tation services are available to private practitioners and health
institutions.
    ● Pediatric Neonatal Emergency Care--A specially equipped
rescue ambulance and a doctor are always available.
    ● Physician Consultation--A speakers' pool, satellite clin-
ics, on-site and WATS line consultation provide increased access
to quality health care services.
    ● Pickup and Delivery Services--Automobile routes covering
over 1,700 miles per day enable pickup and delivery of diagnostic
data and results (i.e., laboratory, X rays, pulmonary functions,
blood banking, and medical equipment needing maintenance or repair
(Marshfield Clinic, n.d.).

    The data documents that the Marshfield Clinic is the dominant
health facility in the Marshfield community and that it has extended its influence into a wide geographical area. In doing so,
it has developed a sophisticated plant and a technological center
that demands high levels of utilization and support. In some ways
it represents a local empire in the health care field. It also
buttresses its position by tying in with and tapping the resources
of the larger society. It has an affiliation with the medical
school of the University of Wisconsin and generates research and
demonstration projects that are supported by the federal government and various foundations.
    The Geisinger Medical Center--The Geisinger Medical Center in
Danville, Pennsylvania, has much in common with the Hunterdon Med-

ical Center and the Marshfield Clinic. It is a sophisticated and
dominant medical establishment located in a nonmetropolitan area.
The Geisinger Center has a 460-bed hospital and 133 physicians in
a closed staff covering almost all specialty areas. The center
functions as a general hospital and family medicine facility for
residents in the immediate area; it also provides tertiary care
on referrals from physicians in central Pennsylvania. The center
has established an HMO (the first in rural Pennsylvania), which
serves an area limited to the county in which the clinic is located.

     More so than Hunterdon or Marshfield, Geisinger Medical Cen-
ter seems to correspond to the model of an empire in the interorganizational field. The position of the Geisinger Clinic in the
field represents an elite center among freestanding hospitals.
Within 20 miles of the center are 6 community hospitals of 100 to
200 beds, which are staffed by community physicians and some general specialists. Farther away are additional hospitals, some in
larger cities such as Williamsport or Wilkes-Barre-Scranton.
These communities have somewhat more tertiary care capabilities,
but Geisinger remains the regional referral tertiary care center
for the area. Geisinger has taken the lead in forming a consortium with 6 of the community hospitals. The field is still one of
competition among units, but clearly Geisinger represents a unit
of strength and one in which the technological imperative leads to
concentration and centralization in operating. For example, 18
member hospitals participated in the Susquehanna Poison Center at
Geisinger, and the neonatal retrieval program, operating in conjunction with the Danville Ambulance Service, retrieved 177 high-
risk newborns from 25 area hospitals (1976-1977) (Geisinger Medical Center, n.d.). The administrators of the center see regionalization in which local hospitals and the center would establish
regular and reciprocal relationships as highly desirable (Hood,
1974). Geisinger, in a manner similar to Hunterdon and Marshfield, is affiliated with university programs of health care and
research, in this case principally with the Hershey Medical School
of the Pennsylvania State University.

Centralization of Control--Toward Corporate Guidance

     Centralization is one of the pervasive developments in medi-
cal services. The imperatives of medical technology and the requirements that accountability of large-scale public financing impose on the system are among the causes of centralization. The
environment of government regulations, threats of malpractice
suits, and requirements of third-party payers are so hostile that
small hospitals need the technical expertise of managers.

Shared services. A significant form of centralization is the
widespread use of professional hospital and nursing home management services. In addition to complete management services, "unbundled" service contracts are becoming common. An unbundled

service is an administrative or clinical service to which a hospital may subscribe while retaining control of day-to-day operations. Among the unbundled services offered are management/purchasing contracts; financial services such as collection, billings, accounting, and auditing; data processing; planning; emergency room services; and alcoholism treatment services. These services may be provided by hospital management corporations, state professional associations and cooperative groups, and hospital chains (both investor-owned and tax-exempt multihospital systems).

Hospital chains are increasing their activities in the unbundled field. In 1979, chains had 2,776 unbundled service contracts with hospitals (44 of the 87 largest multihospital systems offered unbundled services) (DiPaolo, 1979). In 1979, for example, American Medical International of Beverly Hills, California, had 475 contracts and offered 21 different unbundled services. Donald Wegmiller (1978) notes that contract management arrangements are becoming more common where other multiinstitutional arrangements are not readily available to small rural hospitals or when these hospitals are experiencing severe difficulties with finances, personnel staffing, physician recruitment and retention, physical plant planning and development, and other operational problems that cannot be resolved through mere cooperation with neighboring hospitals.

Health Central, Inc., is an organization that has developed a variety of sharing programs and services for rural hospitals throughout a broad region of the United States. It is more comprehensive than many organizations that contract services and it provides a form of regionalization characteristic of a number of hospital chains. Health Central, Inc., is a not-for-profit multiple management service based on six primary member institutions having a total of 1,297 acute and nursing care beds. Three of the member institutions are in suburban Minneapolis, two in small Minnesota towns, and one in a small South Dakota city. Through its programs, Health Central provides shared services to more than 80 hospitals in a six-state region. These include biomedical engineering, accounting and financial services, architectural and engineering services, group purchasing, data processing, management engineering, planning, and public relations (Wegmiller, 1978). In the example of group purchasing, the largest in the upper Midwest, Health Central negotiates more than 250 master contracts, covering 10,000 supply items, with nationwide vendors of hospital products. The participating hospitals purchase directly from the vendors at prices negotiated by Health Central.

Two small rural hospitals in Health Central's ownership system are corporate members. They receive all management services from the corporation and are full participants in the system's corporate decision making and long-range planning. One of these hospitals became a corporate member after being a shared services affiliate for seven years. Wegmiller lists some of the benefits of multi-institutional arrangements; among them are interchanges that are associated with regionalization (the second item below), although compactness of area is not present.

    ● *Savings achieved through greater volume*--Purchasing audits indicated that hospitals could save 20 percent through Health Central's group purchasing.
    ● *Improved accessibility and quality of care*--Through cooperative arrangements, small hospitals can offer their patients and staff members a much wider range of services and greater access to specialists, consultants, and expensive equipment. Staff physicians frequently have staff privileges at all hospitals within a system, so a patient can be admitted by his own physician directly from his local hospital to the referral hospital.
    ● *Greater stability*--Because fluctuations associated with one unit do not have a great effect on the entire system, the system is more attractive to potential financial supporters.
    ● *Political clout*--Because the physicians, trustees, and community representatives of the system serve on boards and advisory committees of health planning agencies, the system's hospitals are able to work more effectively with HSAs.
    ● *Forestalling or eliminating duplication of capital and operational costs*--In many cases cooperative arrangements can eliminate such costly duplication [Wegmiller, 1978].

Presbyterian Medical Services: A case of corporate guidance.
Presbyterian Medical Services (PMS) of New Mexico represents a corporate managed approach to regionalization in which administration is centralized, although local participation is encouraged. PMS serves an isolated area of northern New Mexico. Its information bulletin states:

> PMS operates in a region of great scenic beauty and limited economic activity. Small rural communities of tri-cultural composition (Spanish, Native American, and Anglo) are scattered across a terrain that varies from mountain range to river valley to desert plain. These proud peoples maintain their traditional cultures in small villages and towns largely isolated by distance and hazardous roads from the mainstream of modern society. The region ranks among the poorest in the nation. The median family income for a family of four is significantly below the official poverty level. Living conditions--housing, sanitation, roads, communication--are often primitive. Social services and economic assistance are limited. Access to major medical centers is almost impossible for most of the people of the area.

PMS is a charitable, nonprofit corporation. Its programs are centrally administered and coordinated by a professional staff with expertise in financial management, health care administration, health resources development, and the medical arts. It is an example of a corporate-guided field, which Edward Lehman (1975) regards as a contemporary control configuration because it represents a deliberate response to current problems in the delivery of health services. "It is based on the assumption that the delivery of health services will improve when multiple health care units coordinate their activities under the aegis of a superordinate agency that will administer all of them."

Following a regionalization model, three levels of service are provided: health stations, diagnostic and treatment centers, and hospitals. *Health stations* are very simple facilities located in remote areas of low population. They are staffed by physician assistants and nurse practitioners who maintain radio communication between the stations and the diagnostic and treatment centers. Supervision is provided by physicians located in the diagnostic and treatment centers who make periodic visits to the health stations. The *diagnostic and treatment centers* are more comprehensive ambulatory health facilities. They provide preventive, diagnostic, treatment, referral, and follow-up services. Dental, pharmacy, laboratory and X-ray services, and 24-hour emergency services are also provided at this level. Full-time physicians are located at diagnostic and treatment centers, but extensive use is also made of physician extenders. Much of the technical staff is recruited from the area and represents several ethnic groups. There are two small (under 50 beds) hospitals in the PMS system. They provide secondary level care for people of the area, but tertiary level services are not available within the system.

The system is administered by a professional staff located in Santa Fe. The board of trustees, which directs the overall program, has representatives from communities served by the system, and each of the local units has a local policy guidance council.

Government efforts at corporate guidance. The efforts of state and federal governments to rationalize the health delivery system can be regarded as a form of corporate guidance in an interorganizational field.

The federal government's efforts at rationalization of health services within a regionalization framework can be traced from the Hill-Burton legislation (1946) through Regional Medical Programs (1965), Comprehensive Health Planning (1966), and the National Health Planning and Resources Development Act (1974). These programs have been described in some detail in Chapter Four. The National Health Planning and Resources Development Act has now been in place for some time, and it appears to be more effective than its two immediate predecessors. One of its tools is mandatory state certificate-of-need legislation by which review and approval are made by state agencies of new health facility construction and program expansion above a stated dollar amount. Reviews begin in HSAs and proceed to state level review and final decision.

As building blocks of the health planning system, HSAs have

received the attention of analysts. Jeannette Fitzwilliams (1979)
has specifically considered some of the characteristics and problems of rural HSAs. She points out the wide variability in population size, population characteristics, and physical area of the
nation's HSAs and the need for flexibility in guidelines and regulations.

Almost before the legislation was passed and partly on the
basis of experience with Comprehensive Health Planning (CHP),
questions were raised about local participation, the relative influence of consumers and providers in decision making, and the
relative strength of reviewers and applicants. One of the most
critical and insightful questioners was Bruce Vladeck. He saw the
representation on the governing boards of HSAs as representatives
of numerous interest groups, not as consumers and providers. Vladeck expected log-rolling and reciprocity to prevail in such a
situation. His conclusion was that "the likelihood that (HSAs)
will generate radical changes in the health care system is small.
Rather than conforming to the inspiring exhortations of the pre-
amble to P.L. 93-641, they are more likely to provide an institutional forum for legitimizing existing patterns of power distribution, and to accede as slowly as they can to those irresistible
exogenous forces that would have produced major change in any
event" (Vladeck, 1977). It is of interest to point out that Vladeck's pessimism about HSAs has been somewhat mollified by events.
In another place he says, "The early performance of many HSAs has,
it must be confessed, substantially exceeded the expectations of
many skeptics, including this one" (Vladeck, 1979).

An empirical study was made of participation in the review
process of health programs in Michigan under the CHP program.
This program has implications for HSAs and their review processes.
The analysis was of 260 health facility projects that were reviewed by 19 committees in 10 multicounty "b" agencies. The conclusion reached was that the decision-making agenda of CHP facilities project review is shaped fundamentally by project applicants
and review committees whose recommendations are rarely overturned
by agency governing bodies.

It was pointed out by the author that "while all CHP governing bodies nominally complied with the Federal mandate for consumer control, membership on review committees was generally dominated by providers located close to the meeting, who had even a
greater share of committee attendance" (Faas, 1977). Furthermore,
in the balance between reviewer and applicant, the applicant had
some advantages.

Complex projects presented for review require an investment
of much time and effort by committee members attempting to
understand such projects. The project applicant is usually
well-prepared, being employed as a professional service provider full-time in project activity. As an entrepreneur, the
applicant is in a position to benefit significantly by having
the project approved. In contrast, review committee members

serve on a voluntary basis part-time in project review. Not
only are the costs of organizing opposition to any particular
project high to any individual review committee member, but
the potential collective gain from doing so is widely different among them. Given this unequal incentive structure, the
applicant tends to win against those with nominal control on
the review committee who may not support the proposed project
but cannot sustain an effective challenge against it [Faas,
1977].

Whatever its faults, planning through HSAs has become significant in the delivery of health services. Rural areas in general
are not pressing for new construction of facilities. In many
cases they are concerned with retaining services that under HSA
guidelines are not utilized sufficiently. Most rural participants
in decision making realize that regionalization moves resources
toward central locations and thus from the more rural areas. Rural communities, however, are not without resources in their encounters with regulators and planners of the larger society. This
is illustrated by activities that surrounded building a new hospital in Regionville, a case study in the following chapter.
    A lesson gained from examining federal programs such as Hill-
Burton, Comprehensive Health Planning, and Regional Medical Programs is that they are vulnerable (in ways not applicable to marketplace systems) to change or elimination by decree. Thus planners and analysts cannot be sure that plans and programs will become operational and remain in place. It is likely, however, that
control of the health service system will continue or reappear as
an activity of the federal government, especially in cost containment, and that regionalization in some guise will be involved.

CHAPTER 8

Two Case Studies

Case materials have been used throughout this discussion to illustrate, document, and test concepts and relationships. In this chapter, two case studies are presented to gain a sense of the efforts needed and the multiple factors involved in organizing and implementing community programs. The first case deals with the initiation and development of a community hospital/health center in a nonmetropolitan county, the second with the relationships between a rural community and the agencies of regulation in the building of a hospital.

THE HUNTERDON MEDICAL CENTER

The Hunterdon Medical Center is one of the success stories in rural health care delivery. At the end of World War II, Hunterdon County, equidistant between New York and Philadelphia, was the only county in New Jersey without a hospital. Its economic base was agriculture, with high production of poultry and eggs and a significant dairy industry. The population was about 40,000; Flemington, the county seat and largest city was about 5,000. In 1953, a medical center with a hospital of 100 beds was opened. It was an innovative institution at the time and remains a model for the present. Material in this case is taken from the Hunterdon Medical Center Symposium published to commemorate the center's twentieth anniversary. The authors of the volume (see References) wrote individual chapters.

The discussion that led to the development of the center was initiated by the members of the County Board of Agriculture because of their interest in the health needs of the county. A hospital was proposed as one solution to the problem. At first the Board of Agriculture members were not enthusiastic because no one wanted just another hospital, and a first-class institution was felt to be beyond the county's means (Curry et al., 1974). But, in true committee fashion, the board appointed a study committee to explore the problem. The study committee took its charge seriously, visited other community hospitals, contacted officials, and

151

consulted with the Commonwealth Fund Foundation. The last contact
proved to be especially important in that the Commonwealth Fund
Foundation had experience and interest in innovative community
health projects. It became a source of financial support and informed counsel.

The committee, not satisfied with recommending a minimal hospital and realizing the complexity of their vision, went back to
the Board of Agriculture and obtained funds to employ a consultant. The man employed was E. H. L. Corwin, chairman of the Public Health Committee of the New York Academy of Medicine. Dr.
Corwin was one of the numerous connections to the larger health
services community that played a large part in molding the center.
He had recently participated in the preparation of a report by the
New York Academy of Medicine supported by the Commonwealth Fund.
The report proposed "a new organization of health care delivery,
including a new type of institution that combined a hospital and a
health center" (Curry et al., 1974). The institution would be
community oriented and provide a broad spectrum of health services. The kind of facility and program that Dr. Corwin recommended for Hunterdon followed the report very closely. His design
proposed a hospital in combination with a health center, which
would provide good follow-through social services to the community, and affiliation with a university medical center--"a model of
its kind, able to bring what is best in medicine to the residents
of a rural area" (Curry et al., 1974).

A second element from outside the community that shaped the
center was the New York University Medical School's interest in
developing a regionalized network of hospitals. Under a grant
from the Kellogg Foundation, that institution "inaugurated a regional hospital plan designed to extend to community hospitals in
and around New York affiliation to assist them in providing programs in continuing medical education for their staffs" (Curry et
al., 1974). Among the sites desired was a rural medical center.
In a second report to the study committee, Dr. Corwin specifically
recommended an affiliation with the New York University Medical
School.

A third extracommunity influence in shaping the center was
the recently passed Hill-Burton legislation. In addition to providing a possible source of funding, it required at least minimal
attention to development within a regionalized context. In the
original state health plan under Hill-Burton, Hunterdon County was
divided among the hospital service areas of adjoining counties.

Commentators on the Hunterdon Medical Center from outside the
community are struck with the high level of support by community
members in the undertaking and are perhaps a little surprised at
the sophistication of these rural folk. Fund drives regularly
met their goals without the aid of professional fund raisers. The
community was represented by a board of trustees that consisted of
informed leaders in the community. There had been but one president of the board up to 1974. He was a large-scale dairy farmer
who was chairman of the Board of Control of the New Jersey Depart-

ment of Institutions and Agencies. He received honorary doctor-
ates from Rutgers and Lafayette universities and the Award of
Honor of the American Hospital Association apparently because of
his interest and work in Hunterdon Center.

The national prominence of people associated with the center
is one of the striking things about the Hunterdon story. In the
20 years from 1953 to 1973, the center had four medical directors,
all of whom were at the center in 1953 in some capacity and all of
whom achieved national reputation. For example, Ray E. Trussell,
the first medical director, became Commissioner of Hospitals of
New York City and later General Director of Beth Israel Medical
Center, New York City. The second medical director, Edmund D.
Pellegrino, came to Hunterdon in 1953 as Director of Internal Medicine and became Vice President for Health Affairs and Chancellor
of Medical Units at the University of Tennessee.

Part of the uniqueness of the Hunterdon organization was the
relationship of personnel and facilities offering primary, secondary, and tertiary services. In viewing Hunterdon after 20 years,
Ray E. Trussell said, "In retrospect, as I look back at Hunterdon,
among the many outstanding accomplishments the single most excep-
tional feature has been that of the use of medical personnel of
different degrees of training, goals, and interests and their
working relationships within the same community" (Curry et al.,
1974). Basically, Trussell was referring to the relationship of
primary care physicians in private practice to the hospital specialists.

The medical staff of the center consisted of salaried specialists (the full-time staff) and family doctors in private practice. In 1973, 34 specialists and 25 family doctors were practicing in the community. The specialties represented were internal
medicine (with subspecialties in cardiology, gastroenterology, he-
matology, rheumatology, and metabolic and chest diseases), pediatrics, general surgery (with a subspecialty of vascular surgery),
obstetrics and gynecology, orthopedics, urology, ophthalmology,
anaesthesiology, pathology, and radiology.

Family and general practitioners in private practice were ad-
mitted to the attending staff. Pellegrino described the relationship between family doctors and specialists:

> General practitioners were granted privileges in medicine,
> pediatrics, and normal obstetrics, and minor but not major
> surgery. They admitted patients directly to these services
> and had three options with respect to the specialist staff.
> They could rely on the routine review of their cases by the
> chief of service as part of his daily rounds; they could ask
> for formal consultation with the specialist, retaining their
> role as attending physicians; or they could transfer the pa-
> tient to the full-time staff, resuming care upon discharge.
> Frequent informal consultations between attending general
> practitioners and the specialist staff were essential, espe-
> cially in medicine and pediatrics, where the majority of pa-

tients were attended by general practitioners. In obstetrics, normal deliveries were performed by the general practitioner, but complicated deliveries were the responsibility
of the specialist staff.

Important elements of the professional relationships
were the equal representation on the medical board of community practitioners and full-time specialists; a functioning
professional staff organization that included all physicians,
full-time staff and family practitioners; and effective communications between all physicians, the board, and the medical director. Family physicians were members of all hospital
committees, taking part in teaching and all aspects of planning. Specialists, in turn, were active members of the
county medical society.

Equally essential was the policy in the diagnostic center that specialists should see patients only on referral
from a community physician. Patients were referred back to
the physician promptly, usually with both a personal and a
written consultation report. . . .

The specialist staff, therefore, made a clear effort to
function as consultants, assisting the community physician in
hospital and ambulant care. The generalist in his turn recognized the utility of specialist attention in secondary and
tertiary care. . . .

The general practitioners thus became, from the outset,
an integral part of the total health care system in the
county. The responsibility for primary care was their most
important mission. But they were also the integrating element in the secondary and tertiary levels of care. The benefits to patients were clear. The community had the benefit
of both specialist and family medical care; all levels of
care were coordinated with each other and available in one
community. The only exceptions were the most complicated
problems which were sent to the university centers in New
York or Philadelphia [Curry et al., 1974].

The center extended itself into primary care in two additional ways. It was among the first institutions to offer residencies
in family practice and it developed satellite family practice
clinics in outlying areas of the county. The family practice residency program had 18 positions (6 appointments each year for
three years). Many more applications were received than could be
filled. It is of interest that at the twentieth anniversary most
of the family physicians in private practice in Hunterdon County
(18 of 25) had gone through the center's residency training program.

The satellite family practice program is relatively new. At
the twentieth anniversary of the center, two satellites were in
operation and a third was planned. In one, the staff consisted of
two full-time family doctors on the center's payroll; the other
operating satellite was staffed by two family practitioners in

private practice. In each case, facilities such as social services, physical therapy, laboratories, and X ray were planned to be
phased in. The board of trustees also anticipated that inpatient
beds would be added later.

From its beginning, the center has had formal relationships
with university medical centers and regards the teaching function
as an integral part of its program. The original affiliation was
with the New York University Medical School, which had developed a
regional plan of community hospital affiliations. The relationship was instrumental in staffing the new health center in Hunterdon, and the members of the full-time specialist staff at Hunterdon were on the clinical staff of the medical school. "They . . .
were kept abreast of recent developments by their weekly visits to
teach and learn as members of the faculty of the NYU Bellevue Medical Center" (Curry et al., 1974). Interns from the New York University Medical Center were rotated through Hunterdon and fourth
year students were offered electives at Hunterdon; thus the center
was involved deeply in relationships with a major teaching medical
center. Since 1972, and as New York University became more involved with inner city problems, affiliation has been made with
the New Jersey College of Medicine and Dentistry--Rutgers Medical
School. The degree of cooperation with Rutgers became as high or
higher than it had been with New York University.

In reviewing the development of the center, several things
stand out. One is that an institution was developed that provided
high-quality medical services to a population in a defined area.
A form of regionalization was achieved in which family practitioners in private practice were part of a health care system that
provided secondary and certain tertiary care by a full-time salaried specialty staff within the community. Affiliations with major medical centers, largely through education programs, provided
the expertise of tertiary care both at the Hunterdon Center and in
university medical centers.

A second conclusion is that the form of organization that
developed is not something that some local people stumbled upon.
It is remarkably close to the form suggested by the New York Academy of Medicine's report, *Medicine in the Changing Order*, on which
Hunterdon's principal consultant had worked. The Commonwealth
Fund Foundation was important not only for financial support but
also for advice, especially from the foundation's Dr. Lester
Evans. The chairman of the board of trustees said of Evans, "We
repeatedly turned to him for advice. . . . Certainly he, more than
any other, guided us in those early days" (Curry et al., 1974).
Nor can the community claim financial self-sufficiency in the undertaking. Although local people responded to fund raising
drives, money was also obtained from federal grants and several
foundations.

Also, in spite of nods to the community, the program was professionally designed and controlled. The community was represented in a very traditional way by a board of trustees. This board,
as exemplified by its chairman, was drawn from the community's

elite and was co-opted (not in a negative sense) by the professional system. Community rank and file members might express a sense of community pride and be pleased in a personal sense with the services available, but they appeared not to be closely involved in the policy of the center.

The center monopolized the health care system of the community by incorporating the private practitioners into the system and excluding noncenter specialists through a closed specialty staff in the hospital. Furthermore, the center extended its reach to the more remote parts of the county by establishing satellite family practice facilities. As a facility of substance, it could also deal from strength with organizations outside the community. The leadership was knowledgeable about the health care establishment, including foundations and government bureaucracies. The center offered valued services to the more sophisticated components of the health care establishment as a place for training students from undergraduate through graduate levels. The residency program in family practice was early and successful.

The Hunterdon experience has not been forgotten. Principals in the activity have been reporters as well as innovators and movers. Ray E. Trussell, for example, reported on the experience in a book, *Hunterdon Medical Center: The Story of One Approach to Rural Medical Care* (Cambridge, Mass.: Harvard University Press, 1956), and there are numerous articles in professional journals by participants in the Hunterdon project. The book from which most of this material is taken was the result of a symposium celebrating the twentieth anniversary of the opening of the center. The claim is made in the Foreword of the book that the Hunterdon Center satisfied the recommendation of the Committee on Costs of Medical Care to a remarkable degree, including the formation of group practice and the coordination of medical services with special attention to coordination of rural and urban services. The tone of the symposium was, as one would expect, affirmative.

There was concern, however, with the fact that this successful model had not been widely reproduced. Anne R. Somers, a participant, discussed some of the factors that account for its failure to gain widespread adoption.

• Medical staff opposition or indifference to hospital involvement in primary and/or long-term care.
• The financial bias toward inpatient care still inherent in most existing health insurance.
• The difficult cost bind in which most hospitals find themselves. Hospitals are unable to experiment as they would like with innovative programs, and new ambulatory and outreach programs are the first to suffer.
• The general passion for autonomy by affiliated professionals and institutions.
• The technological mystique as a reinforcement of the disappearing medical mystique (the public gives higher priority to mod-

ern medical technology than to primary care or patient education).
• A totally inconsistent and ineffective federal health policy (Curry et al., 1974).

In spite of the problems that Somers lists, she sees the development of a community health management system with the hospital at its core (similar to the Hunterdon model) as the middle way
and best alternative. The other options are (1) repudiation of
all planning, as well as regulation, and return to a free market
and price competition in the health service industry and (2)
across-the-board federal regulation, with or without some delega-
tion of controls to regional or local authorities. Somers' voice
is influential in health services planning and she has consistently pursued the theme of the hospital as the core of community
health services management, which has the elements of regionalization exemplified by the Hunterdon situation. In this model she
would include HMOs and the American Hospital Association's plan
for community health care corporations. It might be noted in fact
that the Hunterdon Clinic has many of the features of an HMO, differing most radically by not having a prepaid clientele. Efforts
were made to initiate a prepaid program, but they failed.

Finally, in reviewing the development of the Hunterdon Center, it should be observed that the population doubled in 20 years
and became more urbanized. The hospital also doubled in size and
everything connected with the program increased. Under such conditions, it is perhaps justifiable to ask whether Hunterdon has
anything at all to contribute to modeling rural health services.
The counterclaim can be made that initiation and development of
the center took place in a rural county (but certainly not an isolated one). The institution that opened its doors in 1953 had the
elements of the regionalized system in a rural setting.

REGIONALIZATION IN REGIONVILLE

Regionville has special meaning to anyone interested in rural
health. In 1954 Earl Lomon Koos published a book based on a study
of the health behavior of people in this community under the
title, *The Health of Regionville*. It was an influential study in
the developing field of medical sociology. Stephen Kunitz and
Andrew Sorensen returned to Regionville in the early 1970s and
made observations about the health situation and changes that had
taken place. A new hospital opened in 1973 and the authors, in an
unusually detailed account, follow the process from beginning to
end. It is an account that provides insight into the relationships of a community with the multitude of regulatory and planning
agencies--local, state, and national. The tensions with neighboring communities were also depicted as were developing relationships with a metropolitan hospital, which did not turn out in
textbook fashion. In the following pages the details of planning
and building the hospital are presented, taken from the account by

Kunitz and Sorensen in the article, "The Effects of Regional Planning on a Rural Hospital: A Case Study" (Kunitz and Sorensen, 1979).[1]

Regionville is a pseudonym for a town located in the southeastern corner of Regionville County, also a pseudonym. The town has about 5,000 people and the community area about 7,000. Regionville has not changed much in population since 1850 and remains a service center for surrounding rural areas that extend into two adjacent counties. Although Regionville is the largest place in the county, population growth has been greater in the northern part of the county centered on a place referred to as Big Town. Regionville County is regarded as being in the Rochester, New York, region, but the northern part is much more oriented toward that city than is the southern part.

Rochester was a pioneer in hospital planning and coordination. In 1939, six city hospitals were organized into the Rochester Hospital Council, which became the nucleus for the Council of Rochester Regional Hospitals. The council also had support from the Commonwealth Fund and major participation of the University of Rochester School of Medicine and Dentistry. The council covered an 11-county area and among its purposes were to provide financial aid and planning for rational distribution of adequate hospitals throughout the region and to develop desirable and practical joint administrative services. A merger of the Rochester Hospital Council and Council of Rochester Regional Hospitals took place and became known as the Rochester Regional Hospital Council (RRHC). The RRHC had support from the business community, particularly from Eastman Kodak, Rochester's predominant industry. Marion Folsom, an executive of the company, was active not only in local health affairs but also at the state and national levels (he served in the Eisenhower administration as Secretary of Health, Education and Welfare). RRHC also had quasi-official status since many of its members served on the Regional Hospital Planning Council, which was established by the New York State Joint Hospital Survey and Planning Council to review expenditures of Hill-Burton funds.

Marion Folsom, recently returned from Washington, was chairman of the Review and Planning Conference of RRHC and also chairman of the Rochester Hospital Fund drive. Folsom wished to separate the planning function from the other activities of the RRHC. He succeeded in getting the city and county governments, the Community Chest, the Council of Social Agencies, the University of Rochester Medical School, the Rochester Hospital Fund, and RRHC to sponsor the Patient Care Planning Committee (PCPC). When RRHC received federal funds to review the use of Hill-Burton funds, PCPC was delegated the responsibility for the review in Monroe County (the location of Rochester). In the process PCPC became established as a community planning agency.

----

1. Quotations are reprinted with permission of Pergamon Press, Ltd.

New York State, an early starter in health planning, was also influenced by Folsom. In 1964, he chaired the New York State Committee on Hospital Costs, which resulted in the passage of Article 28 of the New York State Public Health Law in 1966. Under this article the Commissioner of Health was empowered to review and approve all health facility construction, alteration, extension, or modification in the state. The mechanism became very important, subsequently, as a certificate-of-need. A companion article (Article 29, known as the Folsom Act) provided for seven regional planning councils for the state, which were to advise the Health Commission through the State Review and Planning Council on applications for construction of new health facilities or extensions of facilities involving capital expenditures of $50,000 or more. Thus New York State had in place a mechanism of review and control of health facility construction that anticipated (indeed modeled) national legislation, which proceeded through Comprehensive Health Planning to the present program identified with the HSAs. RRHC was designated the regional planning council for the Rochester area.

During this time, health planning legislation was also being formulated at the national level. The legislation most relevant to this discussion is the Comprehensive Health Planning Act (PL 89-749) of 1966. The intent of the legislation was to give health planners a degree of control over the organization of health care. RRHC wanted to be designated as a substate planning agency ("b" agency) of comprehensive health planning for the Rochester area and added an "H" to its title, indicating broadened activity as the Rochester Regional Health and Hospital Council (RRHHC). It was challenged, however, by PCPC, which, as we have seen, was a progeny of RRHC. In the process, PCPC broadened its community support and changed its name to the Genesee Region Health Planning Council (GRHPC). In addition to being designated the "b" comprehensive health planning agency for the Rochester area in 1970, it displaced RRHHC as the state review and planning agency under Article 29 of the State Public Health Law. RRHHC was placed on the hospital planning council of GRHPC. This, then, was the "net" of planning and regulatory arrangements that prevailed in the Rochester area during the time that a Regionville hospital was planned and built. In fact, the new legislation and the pulling and hauling among local agencies during the period of construction made the process more complex and seemed to place the hospital plans of Regionville in jeopardy.

Regionville General Hospital was established in 1921, evolving from a small proprietary hospital. Additions were made through the years so that in 1952 it was a hospital of 58 beds. The hospital board consisted of influential community members, including physicians.

In the mid-1960s, one of the leading physicians became concerned about the adequacy of the hospital. In fact, a health service crisis seemed imminent because six of the ten full-time physicians who staffed the hospital had reached retirement age. A

better hospital was seen as one way to attract and retain physicians. The immediate impetus to hospital construction, however,
resulted from a visit from representatives of the state department
of health who were exercising powers of Article 28 legislation.
The visit was to determine the hospital's eligibility for renewal
of its operating certificate under the article. The report of the
department of health representatives was highly critical and indicated major remodeling and updating of equipment would be required before certification would be renewed. The board knew this
was no idle threat, because two hospitals in neighboring communities had been closed.

At this point the hospital board opted for a new hospital,
which they thought could be built for about $2 million, the esti-
mated cost of remodeling. Fourteen months after the visit from
the state health department representatives, a letter was sent to
the state health department by the hospital board stating its intentions. In December 1967, plans for an 80-bed facility had
started through the review process. The first step began with the
Hospital Review and Planning Conference of RRHHC, where preliminary approval was given with the provision that recommendations of
the County Health Planning Committee be considered prior to sub-
mission to the board of directors of RRHHC. At the county level
there were some differences based largely on the north-south division of the county. Regionville was the focus of south county activities, Big Town of north county activities. However, based on
the county study group report, the board of directors of RRHHC in
September 1968 approved the December 1967 letter of intent to the
state health department to build an 80-bed facility. Consultants
were retained by the hospital board to develop plans and in their
report in early 1969 recommended an increase to 85 beds, which
went to the state health department in an amended letter of intent. The estimated cost had risen to $3.4 million.

In June 1969 the hospital board retained an architect and
fund-raising firm to proceed with the development of the new hospital.

> Although plans for the hospital were proceeding now, the
> State Hospital Review and Planning Council's Division of Re-
> view and Planning complicated matters with its staff report
> of October 22, 1969. This report did not suggest that plans
> for the hospital be scrapped, but it raised several questions
> and offered suggestions portending substantial problems for
> approval of the Regionville facility at the next meeting of
> the Review and Planning Council [Kunitz and Sorensen, 1979].

Among the questions raised were: (1) *location of the hospital*--
since the population in the northern part of the county was growing while that in the southern part was stable, it was suggested
that a northern location might be more appropriate; (2) *financial
capability*--reviewing hospital rates and population projections, a
68 percent occupancy rate for 1980 was projected, raising the

question of economic feasibility; (3) *physician manpower*--the age
of physicians in the area was noted and the question was raised
whether new physicians could be recruited; and (4) *definition of
"continuing care" beds*--it was suggested that one way in which occupancy rates would be kept high was to include 30 percent beds
for "continuing care," which might be delivered more economically
in an extended care facility.

These questions, the authors report, raised considerable con-
sternation among the board members since they seemed to threaten
the project; an extended reply was sent to the State Division of
Hospital Planning and Review in less than a month. Of interest,
in considerations of regionalization, is the response on the
question of location.

> The cleavage between the northern and southern sections of
> the county was addressed directly, and it was suggested that
> regardless of population growth, people in the southern end
> of the county were not oriented toward Rochester for either
> shopping or health care. Furthermore, it was pointed out
> that there was massive emotional support for the hospital
> that no population data would be sensitive to: it mentioned
> that the Regionville man on the street "has a kind of pride
> of ownership" in the hospital [Kunitz and Sorensen, 1979].

A new set of hearings then took place under the newly enacted
federal legislation for comprehensive health planning. The Regionville County Comprehensive Health Planning Committee voted
unanimously to support the construction of the hospital and locate
it in Regionville.

> It seems clear at this point that state planners were looking
> at the county as a unit, whereas the county committee members
> saw the southern and northern parts as quite distinct and
> oriented towards different areas. . . . The Regionville mem-
> bers would not give up the notion of having a hospital and
> felt that precedent demanded they continue to have one.
> Moreover, it is clear that they were not willing to compro-
> mise and have the hospital at another location. One inform-
> ant remarked that the Regionville members of the committee
> were willing to fight harder to keep the hospital than were
> other members to oppose them and move it elsewhere [Kunitz
> and Sorensen, 1979].

A new complication involved the GRHPC, which recently had
been designated the substate comprehensive health planning agency
and had replaced the RRHHC as the local state planning agency with
power to review hospital construction under Article 29 of the
state Public Health Law. Kunitz and Sorensen continue the details: "With the development of these powers, the GRHPC staff
person responsible for Regionville County felt justified in again
raising questions about the appropriateness of the planned facili-

ty in Regionville. His questions revolved essentially around the
fact that the hospital as planned was very 'traditional' and no
significant allowances had been made for the provision of ambulatory and emergency care" (Kunitz and Sorensen, 1979). The question of recruitment and retention of physicians was also raised.

At this point in the saga it is not surprising that the GRHPC
staff member who presented these ideas encountered great hostility
from the hospital board, which claimed that the agency only criti-
cized but never helped. Local opposition from other parts of the
area also surfaced, but in spite of questions, GRHPC recommended
approval to the State Hospital Review and Planning Council. It
was now May 1970.

When the authors asked the director of GRHPC why the agency
had approved construction of the hospital when from a planning
standpoint there were several reservations, his reply was, "They
had more data than we did. The consulting firm which they retained was a highly reputable one, and at that time we had no evidence to contradict the recommendations of that firm. So we just
went ahead and gave them what they wanted" (Kunitz and Sorensen,
1979). Further questions were raised about the financial viability of the hospital by the State Housing Finance Agency, which
would be a main source of financial assistance But by this time,
"Although all the legal, economic and planning obstacles were far
from being surmounted, the resistance to constructing the hospital
was gradually being dissipated, and all concerned planning agencies had--at least officially--given solid support to the hospital" (Kunitz and Sorensen, 1979).

The strong desire by both the hospital staff and the Regionville community for relative autonomy in planning and operating
their hospital and their persistence in repeatedly expressing that
desire in the face of resistance from many sources eventually won
the day. According to several informants, another factor contributing to the success of the Regionville hospital board was a combination of political savvy and aggressiveness displayed by some
of the board leaders. "These were 'self-made men' who had built
up reasonably large business firms from simple beginnings with
what one of them described as 'a lot of hard work, refusing to
give up, and a little luck thrown in.' In the course of securing
approval for the new hospital, it was evident that this combination paid rich dividends" (Kunitz and Sorensen, 1979).

While the effort to transit the agency maze was taking place,
the contention for domain within the area and the development of
formal relationships with a hospital in Rochester deserve attention. Even though state health planners tended to view the county
in which Regionville was located as a single unit, ecologically it
was not. The division was between the northern and southern
areas. The northern part of the county was more closely oriented
toward Rochester but locally centered on Big Town. The Regionville area, while not isolated from the metropolitan center, was
the more rural part of the county. The northern part of the
county was in "natural" contention with the southern part. Re-

gionville, however, by virtue of its history, had a claim on the
location of the hospital that could not be easily shaken. The
northerners did complain, however, that emergency services in the
area were not adequate and that the Regionville doctors were un-
interested in their area. During the time Regionville was engaged
in building the hospital, Big Town promoted an ambulatory care facility and explored with a Rochester hospital the possibility of
establishing "satellite hospital beds" at the Big Town facility.
Thus a threat to Regionville was posed by the possibility of its
neighbor developing separate hospital facilities. The financial
contingencies of the new hospital required that it increase its
catchment area. Aggressive physician recruitment was undertaken
and a family medicine group practice was organized in Regionville.
Satellite clinics were established in nearby towns that brought
hospital patients to Regionville. In all these efforts, Regionville attempted to increase its catchment area, and this increased
the use of the hospital, which according to most judgments had
been overbuilt.

The efforts at affiliation between the Regionville hospital
and Highland Hospital of Rochester are perhaps the most direct exhibit of regionalization in the Regionville case. Apparently the
affiliation of a small community hospital and a more sophisticated
metropolitan hospital (Highland Hospital) offered an exchange that
was mutually beneficial. The leading physician in Regionville
felt that affiliation would reduce the provincialism of Regionville physicians and aid in attracting young physicians to Regionville. The advantage for Highland Hospital was that it would monopolize referral of the more serious cases from Regionville physicians and thus increase its occupancy rate. Discussions of cooperation between the two hospitals began. A concrete exchange
took place when the assistant administrator of Highland became the
part-time director of planning for Regionville Hospital (and soon
full-time administrator of Regionville). This administrative support was needed to prepare for licensure and accreditation of the
hospital. In another exchange, residents in the family medicine
program at Highland were used to staff the emergency room at Regionville on weekends. The effect on the Regionville staff was
that they gradually began calling the Highland staff for medical
advice. Although negotiations for affiliation were serious and
partially implemented, interest by Regionville board members and
staff began to cool. The Regionville principals were fearful that
affiliation would lead to merger and loss of local control. The
relationship did not have the advantage that Highland administrators anticipated. Regionville's aggressive recruitment of physicians, including a number of specialists, had been quite successful (perhaps due partly to the developing relationship with Highland). The effect was that more of the complicated medical procedures and treatments could be handled at Regionville Memorial,
and those that could not were likely to be referred to the more
sophisticated university medical center. A general principle
seems to be working here. Increasing the resources of local

health facilities reduces dependency on higher order facilities
and thus interferes with regionalization in the interorganizational sense. Gibson (1977b) also observed this result when more
resources were provided for local emergency medical services, as
did McNerney and Riedel (1962) when rural health centers used
foundation resources intended to promote regionalization to gain
autonomy.

      This case study of the process of planning for and building a
new health facility is instructive in several respects. Local decisions are constrained by local, state, and federal regulations
and regulators. The process of engaging the outside agencies is
political in the down-home sense. Planners have a sense of regionalization and relate local plans to questions of viability,
needs, and some overall idea of a health care system for the area.
The local decision makers are not helpless in encounters with
planning and regulating agencies. There is a strong tendency for
local control that is aided by increasing resources in rural communities. Clearly, the case demonstrates that regionalization is
not revealed by diagrams of location of facilities but is a process of organization.

CHAPTER 9

The Organization of Rural Health Delivery: A Summing Up

Policy in rural health services delivery suffers from a tendency to emphasize the maldistribution of health resources (particularly physician services) and characterize rural society as folk society. Such narrow vision removes from consideration major issues that are transforming health care delivery in the nation. Rural health care delivery must be viewed within the context of the larger society. At the same time, attention needs to be paid to special characteristics of rural society that affect health care delivery.

The sociological issues are organizational issues. In spite of the diversity of rural society, two organizational characteristics distinguish rural from urban society. The first is the relatively greater importance of primary groups and primary group-based social networks in rural communities. The second is the nature of the linkages of rural-based organizations to the bureaucracies of the larger society.

THE MICROORGANIZATION OF RURAL COMMUNITIES

At the microorganizational level, the distinction between rural and urban areas is not the presence of primary groups in the former and their absence in the latter. Rather, primary groups constitute a higher proportion of the social relationships in rural than urban communities. "It is not so much that the city dweller has fewer acquaintances than our villagers, but rather that he has a great many more strangers" (Craven and Wellman, 1974).

The primary group-oriented community provides a social support mechanism that, for reasons involving symptoms of illness and entrance to the sick role, tends to delay, reduce, or avoid use of professional services. Rural/urban differences in utilization of services are as plausibly explained by differences in the microorganization of the respective settings as by differences in physician/population ratios or by differences in values and beliefs.

The microorganizational explanation of differences in use of health services in rural and urban settings might be used to

165

public advantage. Commentators with perspectives as different as
Eli Ginzberg (1978) (economic necessity) and Ivan Illich (1976)
(health improvement) foresee a need for the contraction of level
of professional health services in the decades ahead. The primary
group support mechanism seems especially effective in absorbing
anxiety and stress that lead to professional dependency. It may
provide an alternative to institutionalization through services
rendered by laypersons in the home and is suited through its
socialization capability to change life-styles that increasingly
are recognized as major contributors to illness. In general,
"natural" organizational structures might be the basis for greater
personal responsibility in health care processes. The discussion
in Chapter Three, however, indicates that lay support networks
are fragile and subject to cooptation by the professional health
delivery system. Alford (1975) discusses the relationship of
community interests ("repressed structural interests") to the
established health care interests. He notes that extraordinary
efforts must be exerted if repressed interests are to challenge
dominant interests with any success.

While many more failures than successes of such challenges
have been recorded, one success is Alcoholics Anonymous (AA).
This movement, which incorporates personal-social support, grew up
outside of and as a challenge to the expert system. Originally
deprecated, AA's effectiveness is now widely recognized by the
expert establishment. To its credit, AA has successfully avoided
cooptation.

The possibility exists that "new health practitioners" could
be incorporated into a "community interest" health care system as
an extension of the natural social support network, somewhat as
curanderos in Mexican-American communities. In this case the community would coopt practitioners who are now regarded as extensions of physicians.

Decisions might be made to divert resources from established
health care facilities to activities of the natural community.
For example, resources might be channeled to families rather than
nursing homes for support and care of infirm elderly people and
extended to family- and community-centered hospices rather than
hospitals for terminal patients.

The social nature of sickness, as found in the sick role,
suggests that the definition of nonhealth conditions can be
changed and the means of dealing with them can be altered. As instruments of socialization, as support mechanisms, as legitimiz-
ers of information, primary groups at the microorganizational level would have a central role in such changes. The character of
the microorganization of rural communities suggests greater likelihood of success in such settings.

REGIONALIZATION: LINKAGES OF LOCAL AND EXTRALOCAL ELEMENTS OF
THE HEALTH CARE DELIVERY SYSTEM
While one may hold out hope for the microorganization of the
community as a vehicle for change, it must be acknowledged that

the concentration of resources and the focus of health policy is on the established health delivery system, which incorporates vast resources and commands great power. The main tension is within the system, between control based on a combination of professional and marketplace principles and control based on rational-efficient planning principles. The former is the dominant control mechanism, the latter a present and real challenge. It should be noted that neither of these modes of control would change definitions of disease and illness, the character of the sick role, the means of legitimizing incumbency in the sick role, or the processes of care. They do, however, have implications for the organization of the health delivery system, many of them centered around the concept of regionalization.

The challenge is rationalization of a system, developed without external controls, that fulfills the purposes of equity, quality, efficiency, and comprehensiveness in health care delivery. An attractive response to this challenge is the design and implementation of regionalized health delivery organizations that, through interpretation, can address each of these problems. The need for such organizational mechanisms was advanced by experiences with large-scale personal health care programs such as Medicare and Medicaid and the anticipation of national health insurance. At the forefront of these experiences is the need to contain costs. Much of the national planning effort focuses on this problem.

Regionalization, however, is not the exclusive child of rational-efficiency oriented planners. Those who advocate professional/marketplace controls can cite the "natural" regionalization that has occurred through the orderly location of primary, secondary, and tertiary health services and through professional referral. And they are willing to participate in the planning process through voluntary understandings among unit members of an interorganizational field as a hedge against greater external control.

Viewing the "natural" gravitation toward regionalization, one might conclude that efforts of the rational-efficiency planners toward regionalized health care delivery systems are merely a formalization of relationships that already exist. This is not borne out, however. The difference between unmanaged and managed regionalization can perhaps be best observed by the expected distribution of different levels of services under each mode. According to Christaller's theory of central places based on marketplace principles (unmanaged), services of different levels of specialization are found in centers forming interlocking networks. Centers (and their trade areas) providing lower level services are not satellite to centers providing higher level services but are positioned between three competing higher level centers. Furthermore, trade area boundaries are fluid depending on the economic advantages offered by one place over another.

This is not true with standard plans for regionalization of health services. Boundaries for the entire system are established and lesser service locations are satellite to greater service locations. The relationship is represented by a branching (dendrit-

ic) system or a solar system model. In Christaller's terms, the
interlocking network of central places is based on marketplace
principles, the satellite arrangement on administrative (planning)
principles.

It is the mode of control, however, that best distinguishes
unmanaged from managed regionalization. Voluntary planning may be
regarded as a means of accommodating the apparent deficiencies of
the unmanaged system without changing the status quo of the delivery system. It is the means favored by professional providers
when planning cannot be avoided. Centralized controls, whether
through the ascendency of a dominant unit over an interorganizational field (as in an empire) or through the administration by a
corporate unit, alter the locus of decisions, the concentration of
resources, and style of control. Characteristic of rational-efficiency models, the style of control tends to be bureaucratic.

The delivery system that currently prevails is largely the
result of professional/marketplace factors. One consequence for
rural areas is the much cited maldistribution of services, particularly physicians' services. In the extreme, the most urban category of counties (metropolitan areas of 1,000,000 or more population) has five times as many physicians relative to the population
base as the most rural counties (counties with no urban population). Unrefined comparisons of this type give an extremely distorted picture of the degree of parity between rural and urban
populations. There is no way that one can say that access to physicians is five times greater in the first instance than in the
second. A substantial part of the difference in physician/popula-
tion ratios in rural and urban areas is accounted for by an excess
of specialists in urban areas. But this is to be expected under
conditions of unmanaged regionalization where general services are
closely spaced in minor trade centers and specialized services are
more widely spaced and located in larger centers. It is expected
that persons are able and willing to travel greater distances for
specialized services, and rural people in this country commonly
do. On a trade area basis, both Dickinson (1954) and Fahs and
Peterson (1968) found that most people, rural and urban, were
within a reasonable distance from a physician. The exceptions
were low-density areas. In many of these areas the presence of
physicians is feasible only through economic subsidy. The question is reasonably asked, What obligation does society have to
provide services to people who choose to reside in remote areas?
The problem may be more efficiently solved through mechanisms of
communication and transportation aimed at moving the person in
need rather than providing nearby services. At any rate, the effects of maldistribution of physician services may be overempha-
sized. There is no evidence that the health of rural people in
the United States is jeopardized by lack of physicians in rural
and urban areas. And, as developed earlier, differences in use of
physicians by rural and urban residents may be accounted for as
reasonably by differences in the character of social organization
(primary group networks) as by maldistribution of physicians.

The failure of the professional/marketplace model to meet the needs of rural people seems to be more related to providing appropriate services and continuity in services. The professional model emphasizes having a regular access point (i.e., a family-doctor relationship) and depends on professional referral. Part of the failure of this arrangement to work ideally may be, in fact, a disjuncture between marketplace and professional premises. One can at least note the resourcefulness of people to adjust the professionally advocated mode of behavior to their needs. Thus it is common to seek specialty services directly on the basis of reputation and lay referral, to use emergency room facilities "inappropriately" for primary care services, and to use specialists for primary services--in a sense, to shop around.

The failure to contain costs in providing health services cannot be blamed entirely on the marketplace. More reasonably it should be attributed to mixing an entrepreneurial system with an administration system of third party payments. In it, market constraints are removed by shifting payment to government and employers without adequate means of limiting demand of consumers or charges by providers.

The marketplace/professional system has the advantage of being able to adjust to changing conditions incrementally rather than cataclysmically. In the case of movement of population to the suburbs, physicians and hospitals followed the population with only slight time lag. One might suppose that rural areas might attract more physicians for two reasons The first is the population turnaround, which has produced a greater increase in the rural than the urban population. The second is the substantially larger number of physicians entering practice, including those in primary care. One might expect that rural areas will receive more physicians as their numbers increase. It also seems quite possible that more specialists, especially those offering primary care such as general internal medicine and pediatrics, will be attracted to rural areas.

It can be argued that the fragmentation and overlap that the marketplace/professional system promotes has its own advantages. There is a line of reasoning that maintains that redundancy in social systems is beneficial, even necessary, for the systems' adaptability and survival (Sjoberg, 1960; Terreberry, 1968; Landau, 1969; Zald, 1969). This is the reason that Roland Warren (1971) argues for "interactional field planning," involving a pluralistic health care system, over "centralized out-come planning." The first "encourages competition wherever feasible, intervening only to affect, and occasionally to modify, the interactional field, through differential resource allocation to agencies, rather than through actually seeking to determine agency functions and prescribe agency benefits." The second "attempts through centralized decision-making to allocate resources through master planning so that the optimal distribution of human services is obtained."

Regionalization in the health field is now a term used and

elaborated by planners. To them it does not mean a "natural" interorganizational field characterized by exchanges of specialized,
autonomous units that are ordered by market and professional influences but rather a rational-efficient model of health services
delivery with effective centralized control. Conceptually, there
has been a movement away from the volunteerism of earlier efforts,
which are frequently accused not only of being ineffective but
also of maintaining the status quo. Regionalization, in its more
guided forms, has become a standard model for health planning by
government agencies and by foundations dealing with problems of
health care delivery.
        Regionalization, in its guided forms, centralizes health
services and their control. The means of managing specialized
units is bureaucratic organization. Centralization implies that
service units in rural areas will have a characteristic relationship to the center. This takes the general form of local service
units in relationship with extralocal bureaucratic organization--
the hinterland, vis-à-vis the center. Kenneth Wilkinson (1978)
notes that the shift in economic power from local to regional and
national agencies has created a vacuum in public affairs decision
making in many communities. "Into that vacuum have moved highly
specialized, and often highly motivated and competent agents of
the larger society. Much of the agenda of public action in many
small towns is now set by employees of state and federal agencies.
The result is a more vigorous assault on some public problems than
formerly, but with an emphasis on public relations rather than on
genuine citizen participation." Some see colonialism as a meta-
phor for the relationship, with exploitation of the periphery by
the center. In critiques of centralization, the technological imperative of centralized health facilities is commonly cited. In
this regard, rural areas are similar to the outlying reaches of
the "health empires" of New York City that Barbara and John
Ehrenreich (1971) describe. The requirements of technology (the
latest and the best) drain resources from service areas and research emphasis diverts attention from patients. In the rural/
urban division, rural people may regard centralization as a threat
to local facilities, which are economic props of the community as
well as sources of health services.
        The character of the decision making is apparent in some of
the more successful rural health delivery models such as the Hunterdon, Geisinger, and Marshfield medical centers. These are
thoroughly and professionally organized operations that fit in
the rational-efficiency mold. Their excellence, in fact, is the
reason they dominate if not monopolize the health care services
of their respective areas. In each of the centers the organization and decisions are largely internal to the organization, with
little community participation in policy. In each case, resources of the larger society are tapped by gaining research and
development funds from governments and foundations and by expanding their service areas. It is not surprising that federal programs supporting personal health care such as Medicare and nation-

al health insurance would prefer to deal with health care units
having quality and size similar to these. One attraction of HMOs
is that they constitute units of size and some degree of internal
organization with which national programs can deal efficiently.
     It can be expected that major programs will be cast in the
regionalization framework. The need and challenge is for rural
areas to adjust the programs to the realities and best interests
of rural communities. In this regard, Cordes and Lloyd (1978)
suggest that research should include explicit measures of some of
the more obvious benefits of a network of small hospitals vis-à-
vis a large centralized facility. These benefits include improved access, a more equitable distribution of physicians, and
lower travel costs. The issues of access and travel costs will
take on increasing importance as the energy crisis intensifies.
     It has been shown in a number of instances that rural health
units and rural communities have ability to identify their purposes as separate from the larger system and to pursue their self-
interest. Thus small health clinics in Michigan used resources of
a foundation (intended to promote regionalization) to achieve local autonomy of services instead; a community in Kentucky used the
assistance and program of the university medical school until physicians were recruited to the community, at which point the university program was rejected; the community leaders of Regionville, New York, successfully negotiated the maze of regulations
that might have located their hospital in a more appropriate place
from a regionalization standpoint or might even have eliminated
it. These strategies conform to those recommended by Kornhauser
(1959) to deflect the effects of centers of influence of mass society on individuals. Such efforts, if combined with greater attention to the microorganization of primary groups, might be expected to provide some degree of personal and community control in
a regionalized health care delivery system.

REFERENCES

Ahearn, Mary C. 1979. *Health Care in Rural America.* Washington, D.C.: USDA AIB-428.

Aiken, Linda H.; Lewis, Charles E.; Craig, John; Mendenhall, Robert; Blendon, Robert J.; and Rogers, David E. 1979. The contribution of specialists to the delivery of primary care. *New England Journal of Medicine* 300:1363-70.

Alford, Robert R. 1975. *Health Care Politics.* Chicago and London: University of Chicago Press.

American Medical Association (AMA). 1966. *Meeting the Challenge of Family Practice.* Ad Hoc Committee on Education for Family Practice. Chicago: American Medical Association.

―――. 1976. *Physician Distribution and Medical Licensure in the United States, 1975.* Chicago: American Medical Association.

―――. 1977. *Profile of Medical Practice, 1977.* Chicago: American Medical Association.

Andersen, Ronald; Greeley, Rachel McL.; Kravits, Joanna; and Anderson, Odin W. 1972. *Health Services Use: National Trends and Variations--1953-1971.* USDHEW Publication (HSM) 73-3004.

Bailey, Kenneth D. 1978. *Methods of Social Research.* New York: Free Press.

Battistella, Roger M. 1968. Limitations in the use of the concept of psychological readiness to institute health care. *Medical Care* 6:308-19.

―――. 1971. Factors associated with delay in the initiation of physicians' care among late adulthood persons. *American Journal of Public Health* 61:1357.

Beale, Calvin L. 1978. People on the land. In *Rural U.S.A.: Persistence and Change,* ed. Thomas R. Ford. Ames: Iowa State University Press.

Benson, J. Kenneth. 1975. The interorganizational network as a political economy. *Administrative Science Quarterly* 20:229-49.

Berkanovic, Emile. 1972. Lay conceptions of the sick role.
    Social Forces 51:53-63.
Bernstein, James D.; Hege, Frederick P.; and Farran, Christopher
    C. 1979. *Rural Health Centers in the United States.* Rural
    Health Center Development Series, no. 1. Cambridge, Mass.:
    Ballinger.
Berry, Brian J. L. 1967. *Geography of Market Centers and Retail
    Distribution.* Englewood Cliffs, N.J.: Prentice-Hall.
Berry, Ralph E., Jr. 1973. On grouping hospitals for economic
    analysis. *Inquiry* 10:5-12.
Booth, Alan, and Babchuk, Nicholas. 1972. Seeking health care
    from new sources. *Journal of Health and Social Behaviors* 13:
    90-99.
Bowers, John Z. 1977. *An Introduction to American Medicine--
    1975.* USDHEW Publication (NIH) 77-1283.
Campbell, Angus. 1981. *The Sense of Well-Being in America.* New
    York: McGraw-Hill.
Christaller, Walter. 1933/1966. *Central Places in Southern Ger-
    many,* trans. Carlisle W. Baskin. Englewood Cliffs, N.J.:
    Prentice-Hall.
Clark, Margaret. 1959. *Health in the Mexican-American Culture:
    A Community Study.* Berkeley: University of California
    Press.
Committee on the Costs of Medical Care. 1932. *Medical Care for
    the American People.* Committee on the Costs of Medical Care,
    Publication no. 28. Chicago: University of Chicago Press.
Cordes, Sam M., and Lloyd, Robert C. 1978. Recent social science
    research on rural health services: A critique and directions
    for the future. Paper presented at AMA Conference on Rural
    Health, St. Paul, Minn.
Coward, Raymond T. 1978. Considering an alternative for the
    rural delivery of human services: Natural helping networks.
    Paper presented at annual meeting Rural Sociological Society,
    San Francisco.
Cowen, David L.; Hochstrasser, Donald L.; Friedericks, Carl; and
    Payne, John. 1976. Problems in the development of a rural
    primary care center. *Journal of Community Health* 2:52-59.
Craven, Paul, and Wellman, Barry. 1974. The network city.
    Sociological Inquiry 43:57-88.
Croog, Sydney H., and VerSteeg, Donna F. 1972. The hospital as a
    social system. In *Handbook of Medical Sociology,* 2nd ed.,
    ed. Howard E. Freeman, Sol Levine, and Leo G. Reeder. Engle-
    wood Cliffs, N.J.: Prentice-Hall.
Cumming, Elaine, and Cumming, John. 1957. *Closed Ranks.* Cam-
    bridge, Mass.: Harvard University Press.
Curry, Hiram B.; Henderson, Robert R.; Knocke, Frederick J.;
    Magraw, Richard M.; Millis, John Schoff; Pellegrino, Edmund
    D.; Somers, Anne Ramsay; Trussell, Ray E.; Wescott, Lloyd B.;
    and Wolfe, Samuel. 1974. *Twenty Years of Community Medi-
    cine: A Hunterdon Medical Center Symposium.* Frenchtown,
    N.J.: Columbia.
Daberkow, S. G., and King, G. A. 1977. Response time and the

location of emergency medical facilities in rural areas: A
case study. *American Journal of Agricultural Economics* 59:
467-77.

Dawson Report (United Kingdom Ministry of Health, Consultative
Council on Medical and Allied Services). 1920. *Interim Re-
port on the Future Provision of Medical and Allied Services.*
London: HMS Office.

Decker, Barry. 1977. Federal strategies and the quality of local
health care. In *Health Services: The Local Perspective*, ed.
Arthur Levin. Proceedings of the Academy of Political Science 32:200-214.

Denham, John W., and Pickard, C. Glenn. 1979. *Clinical Roles in
Rural Health Centers.* Rural Health Center Development Series, no. 5. Cambridge, Mass.: Ballinger.

Deutscher, Irwin. 1966. Words and deeds: Social science and social policy. *Social Problems* 13:235-54.

Dewey, Richard. 1960. The rural-urban continuum: Real but relatively unimportant. *American Journal of Sociology* 56:60-66.

Dickinson, Frank G. 1954. *How Bad Is the Distribution of Physicians?* American Medical Association Bulletin 94B.

DiPaolo, Vince. 1979. Forty-four hospital chains see an increase
in unbundled management services. *Modern Health Care* July:
58-59.

Duncan, Otis Dudley, and Reiss, Albert J. 1956. *Social Characteristics of Urban and Rural Communities, 1950.* New York:
John Wiley and Sons.

Dunlop, Burton. 1980. Expanding home-based care for the impaired
elderly: Solution or pipe dream? *American Journal of Public
Health* 70:514-19.

Durkheim, Emile. 1964. *The Division of Labor in Society*, trans.
George Simpson. New York: Free Press.

Ehrenreich, Barbara, and Ehrenreich, John. 1971. *The American
Health Empire: Power, Profits and Politics.* New York:
Vantage Books.

Eisenberg, Barry S. 1977. Characteristics of group medical practice in urban and rural areas. In *Profiles of Medical Practice, 1977*, ed. Sharon R. Henderson. Chicago: American
Medical Association.

Ellenbogen, Bert L.; Hay, Donald; and Larson, Olaf. 1959.
*Changes in the Availability and Use of Health Services in Two
Central New York Counties, 1949 and 1957.* Cornell University
Department of Rural Sociology Bulletin 54.

Ellwood, Paul M., Jr. 1974. Models for organizing health services and implications of legislative proposals. In *Organizational Issues in the Delivery of Health Services*, ed. Irving
K. Zola and John B. McKinlay. New York: Prodist.

Erikson, Kai T. 1976. *Everything in Its Path: Destruction of
Community in the Buffalo Creek Flood.* New York: Simon and
Schuster.

Ewing, Oscar R. 1948. *The Nation's Health: A Ten-Year Program.*
Washington, D.C.: U.S. Government Printing Office.

Faas, Ronald C. 1977. *Decision-Making in Project Review: Proc-*

ess, *Participation and Performance in Michigan Multi-County Comprehensive Health Planning*. Michigan State University Agricultural Economics Report 328.

Fahs, Ivan J., and Peterson, Osler L. 1968. Towns without physicians and towns with only one. *American Journal of Public Health* 58:1200-1211.

Feldstein, Murray S. 1980. Letter to the editor. *New England Journal of Medicine* 302:1034.

Feshbach, Dan. 1979. What's inside the black box: A case study of the allocative politics in the Hill-Burton program. *International Journal of Health Services* 9:313-39.

Fine, Gary A., and Kleinman, Sherryl. 1979. Rethinking subculture: An interactionist analysis. *American Journal of Sociology* 85:1-20.

Fitzwilliams, Jeannette. 1979. *Unmasking Problems in Rural Health Planning*. Washington, D.C.: USDA, Economics, Statistics and Cooperatives Service, Rural Development Research Report 11.

Foley, John W. 1977. Community structure and the determinants of local health care differentiation. *Social Forces* 56:654-60.

Fottler, Myron D.; Gibson, Geoffrey; and Pinchoff, Diane M. 1978. Physician attitudes toward the nurse practitioner. *Journal of Health and Social Behavior* 19:303-11.

Fox, Karl A., and Kumar, T. Krishna. 1966. Delineation of functional economic areas. In *Research and Education for Regional and Area Development*, ed. Iowa State University Center for Agricultural and Economic Development. Ames: Iowa State University Press.

Freidson, Eliot. 1970. *Profession of Medicine*. New York: Dodd, Mead.

Freshnock, Larry J., and Goodman, Louis J. 1979. Medical group practice in the United States: Patterns of survival between 1969 and 1975. *Journal of Health and Social Behavior* 20:352-62.

Fuguitt, Glenn V., and Deeley, Nora Ann. 1966. Retail service patterns and small town population change. *Rural Sociology* 31:53-63.

Galpin, Charles J. 1915. *The Social Anatomy of an Agricultural Community*. University of Wisconsin Agricultural Experiment Station Research Bulletin 34.

Garreau, Joel. 1979. The nine nations of North America. *Washington Post*, March 4.

Gartner, Alan, and Riessman, Frank. 1977. *Self-Help in the Human Services*. San Francisco: Jossey-Bass.

Geiger, H. Jack. 1969. Health center in Mississippi. *Hospital Practice* 4:68-84.

Geisinger Medical Center. n.d. *Geisinger Medical Center Annual Report, 1976-1977*. Danville, Pa.

Gibson, Geoffrey. 1977a. Emergency medical services. In *Health Services: The Local Perspective*, ed. Arthur Levin. Proceedings of the Academy of Political Science 32:121-35.

————. 1977b. Emergency medical services: Regional intents and
    localizing effects. In *Regionalization and Health Policy*,
    ed. Eli Ginzberg. USDHEW Publication (HRA) 77-623.

Ginzberg, Eli. 1978. How much will U.S. change in decade ahead?
    Annals of Internal Medicine 89:557-64.

Glandon, Gerald L., and Shapiro, Roberta J. 1980. *Profile of
    Medical Practice, 1980*. Chicago: American Medical Associa-
    tion, Center for Health Services Research and Development.

Glenn, J. K., and Hofmeister, R. W. 1976. Will physicians rush
    out and get physician extenders? *Health Services Research*
    11:69-72.

Glenn, Norval D., and Alston, Jon. 1967. Rural-urban differences
    in reporting attitudes and behavior. *Southwestern Social
    Science Quarterly* 47:381-400.

Goffman, Erving. 1961. *Asylums*. Garden City, N.Y.: Anchor
    Books, Doubleday.

Goodman, Louis J.; Bennett, Edward H.; and Oden, Richard J. 1976.
    Group Medical Practice in the U.S., 1975. Chicago: American
    Medical Association.

Gore, Susan. 1978. The effect of social support in moderating
    the health consequences of unemployment. *Journal of Health
    and Social Behavior* 19:157-65.

Granovetter, Mark. 1973. The strength of weak ties. *American
    Journal of Sociology* 78:1360-80.

Gregory, Cecil L. 1958. *Rural Social Areas in Missouri*. Univer-
    sity of Missouri Agricultural Experiment Station Research
    Bulletin 665.

Hall, Oswald. 1946. The informal organization of the medical
    profession. *Canadian Journal of Economics and Political Sci-
    ence* 12:30-44.

Hamilton, Horace C. 1962. Health and health services. In *The
    Southern Appalachian Region: A Survey*, ed. Thomas R. Ford.
    Lexington: University of Kentucky Press.

Hampton, Oscar P., Jr. 1976. Categorization of hospital emer-
    gency capabilities: A progress report. *Journal of Trauma*
    16:21-26.

Hardy, William E. 1972. Determination of the Best Locations for
    Rural Health Outreach Clinics: An Economic Analysis Based on
    Virginia Planning District 10. Ph.D. dissertation, Virginia
    Polytechnic Institute and State University.

Hassinger, Edward W. 1957. The relationship of retail-science
    patterns to trade-center population change. *Rural Sociology*
    22:235-40.

Hassinger, Edward W., and Hobbs, Daryl J. 1973. The relationship
    of community context to utilization of health services in
    rural areas. *Medical Care* 11:509-22.

Hassinger, Edward W., and McNamara, Robert L. 1959. *Family
    Health Practices among Open-Country People in a South Mis-
    souri County*. University of Missouri Agricultural Experiment
    Station Research Bulletin 699.

————. 1973. *Changes in Health Behavior and Opinion among Open-*

Country Families in Two Missouri Counties. University of
Missouri Agricultural Experiment Station Research Bulletin
994.

Hassinger, Edward W.; Hobbs, Daryl J.; Bishop, F. Marian; and
Baker, A. Sherwood. 1970. *Extent, Type and Pattern of Medi-
cal Services in a Rural Ozark Area.* University of Missouri
Agricultural Experiment Station Research Bulletin 965.

————. 1971. *Perception of Health Practitioners by People in an
Ozark Area.* University of Missouri Agricultural Experiment
Station Research Bulletin 964.

Hatch, John, and Earp, Jo Ann. 1976. Consumer involvement in the
delivery of health services. In *Rural Health Services*, ed.
Edward W. Hassinger and Larry R. Whiting. Ames: Iowa State
University Press.

Hatch, John W., and Lovelace, Kay A. 1980. Involving the southern rural church and students of the health professions in
health education. *Public Health Reports* 95:23-24.

Hawley, Amos. 1950. *Human Ecology: A Theory of Community Structure.* New York: Ronald Press.

Henig, Robin Marantz. 1976. East Kentucky's answer: A model for
the future. *New Physician* 25:24-27.

Hines, Fred K.; Brown, David L.; and Zimmer, John M. 1975.
*Social and Economic Characteristics of the Population in
Metro and Nonmetro Counties, 1970.* Washington, D.C.: Economic Research Service, USDA, Agricultural Economic Report
272.

Hood, Henry. 1974. *Geisinger Looks to the Future.* Printed
speech at Press Recognition Day at the Geisinger Medical
Center.

Horwitz, Allan. 1977. Social networks and pathways to psychiatric treatment. *Social Forces* 56:86-105.

Ianni, F. A. J.; Albrecht, R. M.; and Polen, A. K. 1960. Group
attitudes and information sources in a polio vaccine program.
Public Health Reports 75:665-71.

Illich, Ivan. 1976. *Medical Nemesis: The Expropriation of
Health.* New York: Pantheon Books.

Johnson, Richard L. 1978. Rural hospitals face change for a
bright future. *Hospitals* 52:47-50.

Kaluzny, Arnold A.; Veney, James E.; Gentry, John T.; and Sprague,
Jane B. 1971. Scorability of health services: An empirical
test. *Health Services Research* 6:214-23.

Kane, Robert; Dean, M.; and Solomon, M. 1979. An evaluation of
rural health care research. *Evaluation Quarterly* 3:130-88.

Kaplan, Berton H.; Cassel, John C.; and Gore, Susan. 1977. Social support and health. *Medical Care* 15:47-58.

Kleinman, Joel C., and Wilson, Ronald W. 1977. Are medically
underserved areas medically underserved? *Health Services
Research* 12:147.

Kornhauser, William. 1959. *The Politics of Mass Society.* Glencoe, Ill.: Free Press.

Kozoll, Richard, and Poncho, Una Mae. n.d. Provision of Material and Child Health Services to a Rural Area--Interaction of a Physician and Physician Assistant in a Rural Health System. Mimeographed paper.

Kraenzel, Carl K. 1953. Sutland and yonland: Settings for community organization in the plains. *Rural Sociology* 18:344-58.

Kunitz, Stephen J., and Sorensen, Andrew A. 1979. The effects of regional planning on a rural hospital: A case study. *Social Science and Medicine* 13D:1-11.

Kupferer, Harriet. 1962. Health practices and educational operations as indicators of acculturation and social class among the eastern Cherokee. *Social Forces* 41:154-63.

Landau, Martin. 1969. Redundancy, rationality and the problem of duplication and overlap. *Public Administration Review* 29:346-58.

LaPiere, Richard T. 1934. Attitudes vs. actions. *Social Forces* 13:230-37.

Larson, Olaf F. 1978. Values and beliefs of rural people. In *Rural U.S.A.: Persistence and Change,* ed. Thomas R. Ford. Ames: Iowa State University Press.

Larson, Olaf F., and Rogers, Everett M. 1964. Rural society in transition: The American setting. In *Our Changing Rural Society: Perspectives and Trends,* ed. James H. Copp. Ames: Iowa State University Press.

Lee, Richard C. 1979. Designation of health manpower shortage areas for use by public health service programs. *Public Health Reports* 94:48-59.

Lehman, Edward W. 1975. *Coordinating Health Care: Explorations in Interorganizational Relations.* Beverly Hills and London: Sage Publications.

Levin, Lowell S.; Katz, Alfred H.; and Holst, Erik. 1976. *Self-Care: Lay Initiatives in Health.* New York: Prodist.

Levine, Sol, and Kozloff, Martin A. 1978. The sick role: Assessment and overview. *American Review of Sociology* 4:317-43.

Levine, Sol, and White, Paul E. 1961. Exchange as a conceptual framework for the study of interorganizational relationships. *Administrative Science Quarterly* 5:583-601.

Levine, Sol; White, Paul E.; and Paul, Benjamin D. 1963. Community interorganizational problems in providing medical care and social services. *American Journal of Public Health* 53:1183-93.

Leyes, John M.; Miller, J. Stuart; Lofgren, Joyce; White, Jeffrey; and Goetz, Sara. 1973. *The Delineation of Economic and Health Service Areas and the Location of Health Manpower Education Programs.* Laramie: University of Wyoming.

Liebow, Elliot. 1967. *Tally's Corner: A Study of Negro Street-corner Men.* Boston: Little, Brown.

Lin, Nan; Simeone, Ronald S.; Ensel, Walter M.; and Kuo, Wen.

1979. Social support, stressful life events, and illness: A model and empirical test. *Journal of Health and Social Behavior* 20:108-19.

Lionberger, Herbert F. 1960. *Adoption of New Ideas and Practices.* Ames: Iowa State University Press.

Litwak, Eugene, and Hylton, Lydia F. 1962. Interorganizational analysis: A hypothesis on coordinating agencies. *Administrative Science Quarterly* 6:395-426.

Lloyd, Peter E., and Dicken, Peter. 1972. *Location in Space: A Theoretical Approach to Economic Geography.* New York: Harper and Row.

Lowe, George D., and Peek, Charles W. 1974. Location and lifestyle: The comparative explanatory ability of urbanism and rurality. *Rural Sociology* 39: 392-420.

Luft, Harold S. 1980. Assessing the evidence on HMO performance. *Milbank Memorial Fund Quarterly: Health and Society* 58:501-36.

Luft, Harold S.; Hershey, John C.; and Morrell, Joan. 1976. Factors affecting the use of physician services in a rural community. *American Journal of Public Health* 66:865-71.

Luft, Harold; Bunker, John; and Enthoven, Alain C. 1979. Should operations be regionalized? The empirical relation between surgical volume and mortality. *New England Journal of Medicine* 301:1364-69.

McCorkle, Thomas. 1961. Chiropractic: A deviant theory of disease and practice in contemporary western culture. *Human Organization* 20:20-22.

McKinlay, John B. 1973. Social networks, lay consultation and help-seeking behavior. *Social Forces* 51:275-92.

McNerney, Walter J., and Riedel, Donald C. 1962. *Regionalization and Rural Health Care.* University of Michigan, Graduate School of Business Administration, Bureau of Hospital Administration.

Madison, Donald L., and Shenkin, Budd N. 1980. Preparing to serve--NHSC scholarships and medical education. *Public Health Reports* 95:3-8.

Madsen, William. 1964. *Mexican-Americans of the Southwest.* New York: Holt, Rinehart and Winston.

Magnuson, Paul B., chairman. 1952. *The President's Commission on the Health Needs of the Nation.* Washington, D.C.: U.S. Government Printing Office.

Marshfield Clinic. n.d. The Marshfield Clinic for the One in Four. Information bulletin of the Marshfield Clinic. Marshfield, Wis.

Martinez, Cervando, Jr. 1977. Curanderos: Clinical aspects. *Journal of Operational Psychiatry* 8:35-38.

Metropolitan Life Insurance Co. 1978. Metropolitan Life Insurance Statistical Bulletin 59.

Miller, Michael K., and Crader, Kelly W. 1979. Rural-urban differences in two dimensions of community satisfaction. *Rural Sociology* 44:489-504.

Moore, Dan E.; Taietz, Philip; and Young, Frank W. 1974. Loca-
    tion of institutions in upstate New York. *Search* 4:1-7.
Morgan, Bruce B., and McKim, Robert L., Jr. 1976. *Rural Health
    Delivery in the Midwest*. Kansas City, Mo.: Midwest Research
    Institute Report for Farmland Industries.
Moscovice, Ira, and Rosenblatt, Roger. 1979. The viability of
    mid-level practitioners in isolated rural communities. *Amer-
    ican Journal of Public Health* 69:503-5.
Mott, Basil J. F. 1968. *Anatomy of a Coordinating Council*.
    Pittsburgh: University of Pittsburgh Press.
————. 1971. Coordination and inter-organizational relations in
    health. In *Interorganizational Research in Health: Confer-
    ence Proceedings*, ed. Paul E. White and George J. Vlasak.
    Washington, D.C.: U.S. Government Printing Office.
————. 1977. The new health planning system. In *Health Serv-
    ices: The Local Perspective*, ed. Arthur Levin. Proceedings
    of the Academy of Political Science 32:238-56.
Mountin, Joseph W.; Pennell, Elliott H.; and Hoge, Vane M. 1945.
    *Health Services Areas: Requirements for General Hospitals
    and Health Centers*. United States Public Health Service Bul-
    letin 292.
Mullan, Fitzhugh. 1980. Physicians for the underserved. *Public
    Health Reports* 95:9-11.
Mynko, Lizabeth Fay. 1974. Health and Illness in Rural America.
    Ph.D. dissertation, Ohio State University.
Nall, Frank, and Speilberg, Joseph. 1967. Social and cultural
    factors in responses of Mexican-Americans to medical treat-
    ment. *Journal of Health and Social Behavior* 8:299-308.
National Center for Health Statistics. 1974. Health characteris-
    tics by geographic region, large metropolitan areas and other
    places of residence, United States, 1969-70. *Vital and
    Health Statistics*, ser. 10, no. 86. Washington, D.C.:
    USDHEW.
————. 1979. Physician visits: Volume and interval since last
    visit. *Vital and Health Statistics*, ser. 10, no. 128. Wash-
    ington, D.C.: USDHEW.
National Commission on Community Health Services. 1966. *Health
    Is a Community Affair*. Cambridge, Mass.: Harvard University
    Press.
Nelkin, Dorothy, and Edelman, David J. 1976. Centralizing health
    care. *Society* 13:26-33.
Nooe, Roger. 1980. Deinstitutionalization in rural areas. *Human
    Services in the Rural Environment* 5:17-20.
Odum, Howard W. 1936. *Southern Regions of the United States*.
    Chapel Hill: University of North Carolina Press.
Orcutt, James D., and Cairl, Richard E. 1979. Social definitions
    of the alcoholic: Reassessing the importance of imputed re-
    sponsibility. *Journal of Health and Social Behavior* 20:290-
    95.
Ostow, Miriam, and Brudney, Karen. 1977. Regional medical pro-

grams. In *Regionalization and Health Policy*, ed. Eli Ginz-
    berg. USDHEW Publication (HRA) 77-623.
Parsons, Talcott. 1951. *The Social System*. Glencoe, Ill.: Free
    Press.
Pearson, David A. The concept of regionalization of personal
    health services in the United States, 1920-1955. In *The Re-
    gionalization of Personal Health Services*, ed. Everett
    Saward. New York: Prodist.
Peters, Ann D., and Chase, Charles L. 1967. Patterns of health
    care in a rural southern county. *American Journal of Public
    Health* 57:409-23.
Pratt, Lois. 1976. *Family Structures and Effective Health Behav-
    ior: The Energized Family*. Boston: Houghton-Mifflin.
Quesada, Gustavo, and Heller, Peter L. 1977. Sociocultural bar-
    riers to medical care among Mexican Americans in Texas. *Med-
    ical Care* 15:93-101.
Raper, Arthur. 1943. *Tenants of the Almighty*. Chapel Hill:
    University of North Carolina Press.
Roebuck, Julian, and Cowie, James B. 1975. *An Ethnography of a
    Chiropractic Clinic: Definitions of a Deviant Situation*.
    New York: Free Press.
Roemer, Milton I. 1976a. Historical perspective of health serv-
    ices in rural America. In *Rural Health Services: Organiza-
    tion, Delivery, and Use*, ed. Edward W. Hassinger and Larry R.
    Whiting. Ames: Iowa State University Press.
————. 1976b. The international experience. In *The Regionali-
    zation of Personal Health Services*, ed. Ernest W. Saward.
    New York: Prodist.
Roemer, Ruth; Frank, Jeanne; and Kramer, Charles. 1975. *Planning
    Urban Health Services: From Jungle to System*. New York:
    Springer.
Rogers, Everett M., and Shoemaker, F. Floyd. 1971. *Communication
    of Innovation: A Cross-Cultural Approach*. New York: Free
    Press.
Rosenblatt, Roger A., and Moscovice, Ira. 1978. Establishing new
    rural practices: Some lessons from a federal experience.
    Journal of Family Practice 7:755-63.
Ross, Peggy J.; Bluestone, Herman; and Hines, Fred K. 1979. In-
    dicators of Social Well-Being for U.S. Counties. USDA Rural
    Development Research Report 10.
Rubel, Arthur J. 1966. *Across the Tracks: Mexican-Americans in
    a Texas City*. Austin: University of Texas Press.
Rural Practice Project. 1976. *Program Bulletin: The Administra-
    tor*. University of North Carolina School of Medicine, Chapel
    Hill.
Rushing, William A. 1975. *Community, Physicians and Inequality:
    A Sociological Study of the Maldistribution of Physicians*.
    Lexington, Mass.: D. C. Heath.
Salber, Eva J. 1979. The lay advisor as a community health re-
    source. *Journal of Health Politics, Policy and Law*. 3:469-
    78.

Salloway, Jeffrey C., and Dillon, Patrick B. 1973. A comparison of family networks and friend networks in health care utilization. *Journal of Comparative Family Studies* 4:131-42.

Sauer, Herbert I. 1976. Risk of illness and death in metropolitan and nonmetropolitan areas. In *Rural Health Services: Organization, Delivery, and Use*, ed. Edward W. Hassinger and Larry R. Whiting. Ames: Iowa State University Press.

Saunders, Lyle. 1954. *Cultural Differences and Medical Care: The Case of the Spanish-Speaking People of the Southwest*. New York: Russell Sage Foundation.

Segall, Alexander. 1976. The sick role concept: Understanding illness behavior. *Journal of Health and Social Behavior* 17: 162-69.

Selznick, Philip. 1953. *TVA and the Grass Roots, A Study in the Sociology of Formal Organization*. Berkeley: University of California Press.

Shannon, Gary W., and Dever, G. E. Alan. 1974. *Health Care Delivery: Spatial Perspectives*. New York: McGraw-Hill.

Sheps, Cecil G., and Bachar, Miriam. 1981. Rural areas and personal health services: Current strategies. *American Journal of Public Health* 71:77-82.

Shevky, Eshref, and Bell, Wendell. 1955. *Social Area Analysis: Theory, Illustrative Application and Computational Procedures*. Stanford, Calif.: Stanford University Press.

Shevky, Eshref, and Williams, Marilyn. 1949. *The Social Areas of Los Angeles: Analysis and Typology*. Berkeley: University of California Press.

Shortell, Stephen. 1973. Patterns of referral among internists in private practice: A social exchange model. *Journal of Health and Social Behavior* 14:335-47.

Sjoberg, Gideon. 1960. Contradictory functional requirements and social systems. *Journal of Conflict Resolution* 4:198-208.

Smith, Carol A. Regional economic systems: Linking geographical models and socioeconomic problems. In *Regional Analysis*, 2 vols., ed. Carol A. Smith. New York: Academic Press.

Somers, Anne R. 1971a. Ameriplan/HCC/HMO--Call it anything, but the hospital is the system. *Modern Hospital* 116:47-48.

————. 1971b. *Health Care in Transition, Directions for the Future*. Chicago: Health Research and Education Trust.

Stam, Jerome M. 1979. Office of Management and Budget, Circular A-95: An Overview. Staff Paper, Economic, Statistics, and Cooperative Services, USDA.

Stevens, Rosemary. 1977. Health manpower. In *Regionalization and Health Policy*, ed. Eli Ginzberg. USDHEW Publication (HRA) 77-623.

Suchman, Edward A. 1964. Sociomedical variations among ethnic groups. *American Journal of Sociology* 60:319-31.

————. 1965. Social patterns of illness and medical care. *Journal of Health and Human Behavior* 6:2-16.

Suttles, Gerald. 1968. *The Social Order of the Slum: Ethnicity*

and Territory in the Inner City. Chicago and London: University of Chicago Press.

Taietz, Philip. 1973. Structural complexity of New York State
communities: Health and welfare. *Search* 2:1-15.

Terreberry, Shirley. 1968. The evolution of organizational environments. *Administrative Science Quarterly* 12:590-613.

Twaddle, Andrew C., and Hessler, Richard M. 1977. *A Sociology of
Health.* St. Louis, Mo.: C. V. Mosby.

Udy, Stanley, Jr. 1958. Bureaucratic elements in organizations:
Some research findings. *American Sociological Review* 23:415-
17.

U.S. Bureau of the Census. 1978. *Statistical Abstract of the
United States: 1978,* 99th ed. Washington, D.C.: U.S. Government Printing Office.

U.S. Department of Health, Education and Welfare (USDHEW). 1976a.
*The Area Resource File: A Manpower Planning and Research
Tool.* Washington, D.C.: U.S. Government Printing Office.

————. 1976b. *Health--United States, 1975.* USDHEW Publication
(HRA) 76-1232.

————. 1978a. *National Guidelines of Health Planning.* USDHEW
Publication (HRA) 78-643.

————. 1978b. *Program Guidance Material for the RHI, UHI, and
HNSC.* Rockville, Md.: Public Health Service, Health Services Administration, Bureau of Community Health Services.

————. 1980. *Health--United States, 1979.* USDHEW Publication
(PHS) 80-1232.

Vance, Rupert B. 1929. *Human Factors in Cotton Culture.* Chapel
Hill: University of North Carolina Press.

————. 1968. Region. In *International Encyclopedia of the Social Sciences,* vol. 13, ed. David L. Sills. New York:
Macmillan, Free Press.

Vidich, Arthur J., and Bensman, Joseph. 1958. *Small Town in Mass
Society.* Princeton, N.J.: Princeton University Press.

Vladeck, Bruce. 1977. Interest group representation and the
HSA's: Health planning and political theory. *American Journal of Public Health* 67:23-29.

————. 1979. Health planning--Participation and its discon-
tents. *American Journal of Public Health* 69:331-32.

Warren, Roland L. 1971. Alternative strategies in interagency
planning. In *Interorganizational Research in Health: Conference Proceedings,* ed. Paul E. White and George J. Vlasak.
Washington, D.C.: U.S. Government Printing Office.

————. 1978. *The Community in America,* 3rd ed. Chicago: Rand
McNally.

Warren, Roland L.; Rose, Stephen M.; and Bergunder, Ann F. 1974.
The Structure of Urban Reform. Lexington, Mass.: D. C.
Heath.

Weaver, Jerry L. 1973. Mexican-American health care behavior: A
cultural review of the literature. *Social Science Quarterly*
54:85-102.

Webb, Walter Prescott. 1936. *The Great Plains*. Boston: Houghton Mifflin.

Wegmiller, Donald C. 1978. Multi-institutional pacts offer rural hospitals do-or-die options. *Hospitals* 52:51-54.

Weisenberg, Matisyohu; Kegeles, S. Stephen; and Lund, Adrian K. 1980. Children's health beliefs and acceptance of a dental preventive activity. *Journal of Health and Social Behavior* 21:59-74.

Weller, Jack E. 1965. *Yesterday's People: Life in Contemporary Appalachia*. Lexington: University of Kentucky Press.

Werko, L. Sevedish. 1971. Medical care in transition. *New England Journal of Medicine* 284:360-66.

West, James. 1945. *Plainville, U.S.A.* New York: Columbia University Press.

Whyte, William F. 1943. *Street Corner Society: The Social Structure of an Italian Slum*. Chicago: University of Chicago Press.

Wilkinson, Kenneth P. 1978. Rural community change. In *Rural U.S.A.: Persistence and Change*, ed. Thomas R. Ford. Ames: Iowa State University Press.

Yordy, Karl D. Regionalization of health services: Current legislative directions in the United States. In *The Regionalization of Personal Health Services*, ed. Ernest W. Saward. New York: Prodist.

Young, Frank W., and Young, Ruth C. 1973. *Comparative Studies of Community Growth: Rural Sociological Society Monograph*, no. 2. Morgantown: West Virginia University.

Zald, Mayer N. 1969. The structure of society and social service integration. *Social Science Quarterly* 50:557-67.

Zook, Christopher J., and Moore, Francis D. 1980. High-cost users of medical care. *New England Journal of Medicine* 302:996-1002.

INDEX

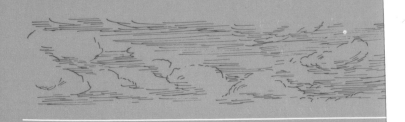

RURAL HEALTH ORGANIZATION: Social Networks and R[egionaliza]tion looks at the problems of rural health services within the [organiza]tional context of contemporary rural society, discussing c[urrent pro]grams as well as future trends. The book considers the c[haracteris]tics and effects of regionalization on the delivery of healt[h services] and explores the effects of personal social networks on uti[lization of] health services.

Edward W. Hassinger places rural health services in a [geographi]cal and a societal context in *Rural Health Organization*. He [examines] the organization of rural health services at two levels. The [first is the] microorganization level, which relates the characteristics [of small-] group networks to decisions about use of rural health servi[ces and as] used as a resource in obtaining health services. The seco[nd level is] the macroorganization level, in which Hassinger considers [regionaliza]tion and regionalization of health services.

Hassinger provides a fresh approach to an old proble[m, applies a] sociological perspective to the problem of health delivery, a[nd organizes] a large amount of information in a conceptual framework.

IOWA STATE UNIVERSITY PRESS ● AMES, IO[WA]

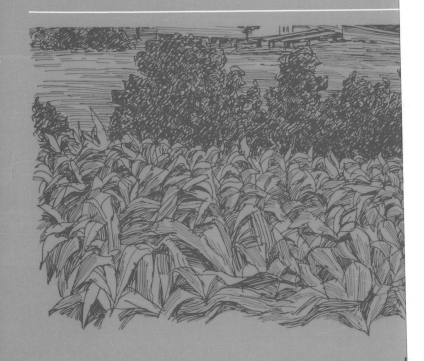